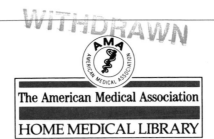

The American Medical Association
HOME MEDICAL LIBRARY

THE RESPIRATORY SYSTEM

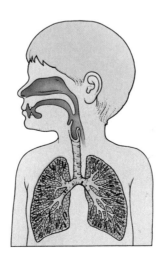

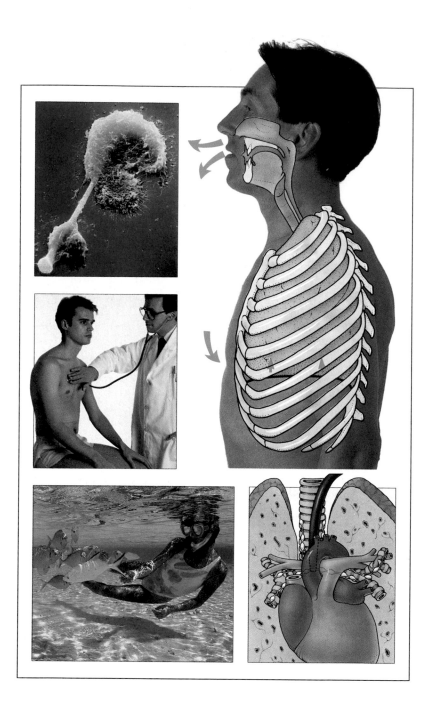

THE AMERICAN
MEDICAL ASSOCIATION

THE
RESPIRATORY
SYSTEM

Medical Editor
CHARLES B. CLAYMAN, MD

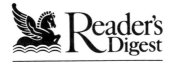

THE READER'S DIGEST ASSOCIATION, INC.
Pleasantville, New York/Montreal

The information in this book reflects current medical knowledge. The
recommendations and information are appropriate in most cases;
however, they are not a substitute for medical diagnosis. For specific
information concerning your personal medical condition, the AMA
suggests that you consult a physician.

The names of organizations, products, or alternative therapies appearing
in this book are given for informational purposes only. Their inclusion
does not imply AMA endorsement, nor does the omission of any
organization, product, or alternative therapy indicate AMA disapproval.

The AMA Home Medical Library is distinct from and unrelated to the
series of health books published by Random House, Inc., in conjunction
with the American Medical Association under the names "The AMA Home
Reference Library" and "The AMA Home Health Library."

Library of Congress Cataloging in Publication Data

The Respiratory system / medical editor, Charles B. Clayman.
      p.   cm. — (The American Medical Association home medical
library)
   At head of title: The American Medical Association.
   Includes index.
   ISBN 0-89577-440-2
   1. Respiratory organs—Diseases. 2. Respiratory organs— Popular
works. I. Clayman, Charles B. II. American Medical Association.
III. Series.
   [DNLM: 1. Respiration Disorders—popular works. 2. Respiratory
System—physiology—popular works. 3. Smoking—adverse effects—
popular works.   WF   100 R434]
RC731.R49 1992
616.2—dc20
DNLM/DLC
for Library of Congress   92-11718

FOREWORD

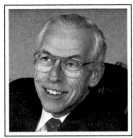

Breathing is the most fundamental expression of life. But breathing is only a part of the complex process called respiration. This process begins when you inhale air. Deep inside your lungs, the oxygen contained in air passes into your bloodstream. Carbon dioxide, a waste product made in your cells, passes from your blood into your lungs so you can get rid of it when you exhale. Your blood transports the oxygen to your body's cells, which need it to produce energy from the food you eat. Respiration encompasses this entire series of events.

In this volume of the AMA Home Medical Library, we describe the workings of the respiratory system in terms you can easily understand. The opening chapter explains the structure of your respiratory system and its function in your body. Later chapters discuss respiratory system disorders – from the common cold to lung cancer. We describe how your doctor diagnoses and treats such disorders and the steps you can take to prevent them.

The most important threat to respiratory health is tobacco smoking, which claims thousands of lives each year from chronic bronchitis, emphysema, and lung cancer. This volume describes how tobacco compromises a smoker's health and the health of others. It also provides information to help you, or someone you know, stop smoking. This book also covers environmental and occupational hazards to respiratory health, which can cause disease years after the person's exposure to them. Poor air quality can also irritate sensitive airways and worsen such conditions as asthma.

We at the American Medical Association hope this volume increases your understanding of the respiratory system and helps you learn how to keep it healthy for your entire life.

James S Todd MD

JAMES S. TODD, MD
Executive Vice President
American Medical Association

THE AMERICAN
MEDICAL ASSOCIATION

CONTENTS

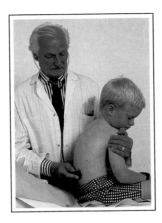

CHAPTER ONE

THE BREATH OF LIFE

INTRODUCTION

WHAT IS
RESPIRATION?

THE BREATHING
PLANET

YOUR
RESPIRATORY
TRACT

YOUR LUNGS

HOW YOUR
BLOOD
TRANSPORTS
OXYGEN

BREATHING

IN 1771, SWEDISH CHEMIST Karl Wilhelm Scheele discovered that an invisible, odorless gas was present in air. Scheele recognized that the previously unknown element was essential both for life and for the burning of a flame. But by the time Scheele described his work on the gas he called "fire air" in a book published in 1777, English chemist Joseph Priestley had reported his own similar experiments and had already taken credit for the discovery of the gas we now call oxygen. Neither Scheele nor Priestley fully understood the role this gas plays in the combustion of fuel or in the body's production of energy. Then, in 1779, French chemist Antoine Lavoisier asserted that air contained two gases. One gas was essential for combustion and the other was not. He called the gas needed for combustion oxygen and the other gas nitrogen. Just as a flame needs oxygen to burn, every cell in your body needs oxygen to "burn" fuel in the form of glucose, a simple sugar derived from the food you eat. This combustion of fuel is the way that every cell in your body obtains the energy it needs to function. Some cells in your body, such as the nerve cells in your brain, depend so heavily on their supply of oxygen that cutting it off for only a few minutes causes permanent damage.

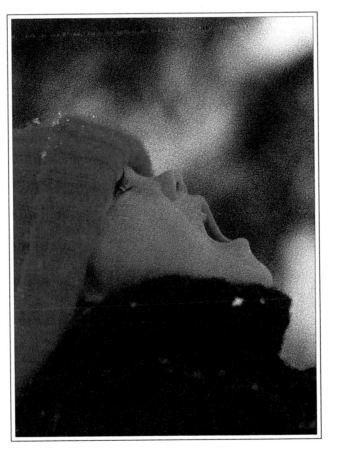

Your cells derive this vital supply of oxygen from the air you breathe and use it to produce energy during a process called respiration. Simple, single-celled organisms can obtain oxygen directly from the atmosphere through their cell membranes. But the human body consists of billions of cells, most of which are not in direct contact with the atmosphere. Your respiratory system is the elaborate structure that transports oxygen to the individual cells in your body. This system consists of your nose; throat; larynx; windpipe (trachea); lungs, containing small air tubes (bronchi and bronchioles) and millions of air spaces (alveoli); and a system of arteries, veins, and smaller vessels that carry blood to and from the lungs. The blood transports nutrients, hormones, antibodies, and waste products around your body, but the most vital function of your blood is the transport of oxygen from your lungs to the fluid that surrounds the cells in your body. The respiratory system also rids your body of the principal waste product of glucose combustion – carbon dioxide. The blood carries this compound from your body's cells to your lungs, so you can expel it when you exhale. This chapter describes the respiratory process and explains how your body performs this complex and essential function.

WHAT IS RESPIRATION?

Many people think respiration has the same meaning as breathing, but this assumption is not quite accurate. Scientists define respiration as the entire process by which oxygen reaches your body's cells and is used by them to produce energy. Breathing, one part of the process, is simply the means by which air enters and leaves your lungs. Respiration is an essential process because you need energy to perform any action. This energy comes from the food you eat. But the energy must be freed from the food before your cells can use it. Respiration includes the process that frees energy so it can be used by your cells.

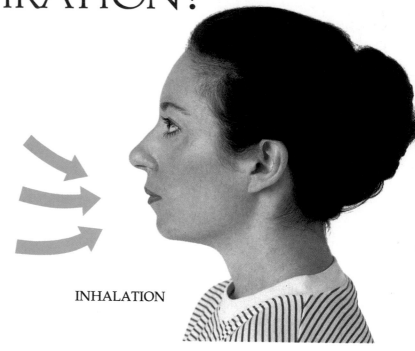

INHALATION

RESPIRATION

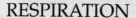

Respiration includes two different processes – external respiration and internal respiration. During external respiration, you inhale air and your blood absorbs oxygen from it. When you exhale, carbon dioxide returns to the atmosphere. Internal respiration refers to the exchange of oxygen and carbon dioxide between the cells of your body and your blood and to the use of oxygen by your cells.

Rod-shaped or cylindrical cell substructures called mitochondria serve as the site of respiration. They are the "powerhouses" of the cell's activities. These energy-producing structures contain enzymes that, in the presence of oxygen, break down glucose derived from carbohydrates in the food you eat to release energy. The number of mitochondria in each cell varies depending on the cell's size and energy expenditure. For example, a muscle cell needs more mitochondria than a skin cell because a muscle cell expends more energy.

RESPIRATION EQUATION

Energy produced in your cells by chemical reaction fuels every action that you perform. When glucose and oxygen react in your cells to form energy, they release carbon dioxide and water as waste products.

Cells can also produce energy for a short time without oxygen. But this process leads to an "oxygen debt" – the accumulation of substances that must later be broken down in the presence of oxygen.

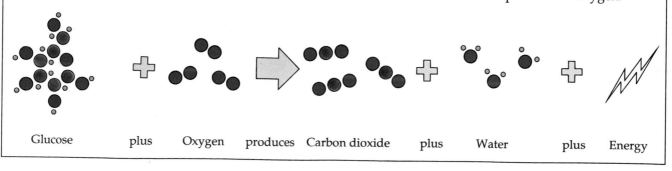

| Glucose | plus | Oxygen | produces | Carbon dioxide | plus | Water | plus | Energy |

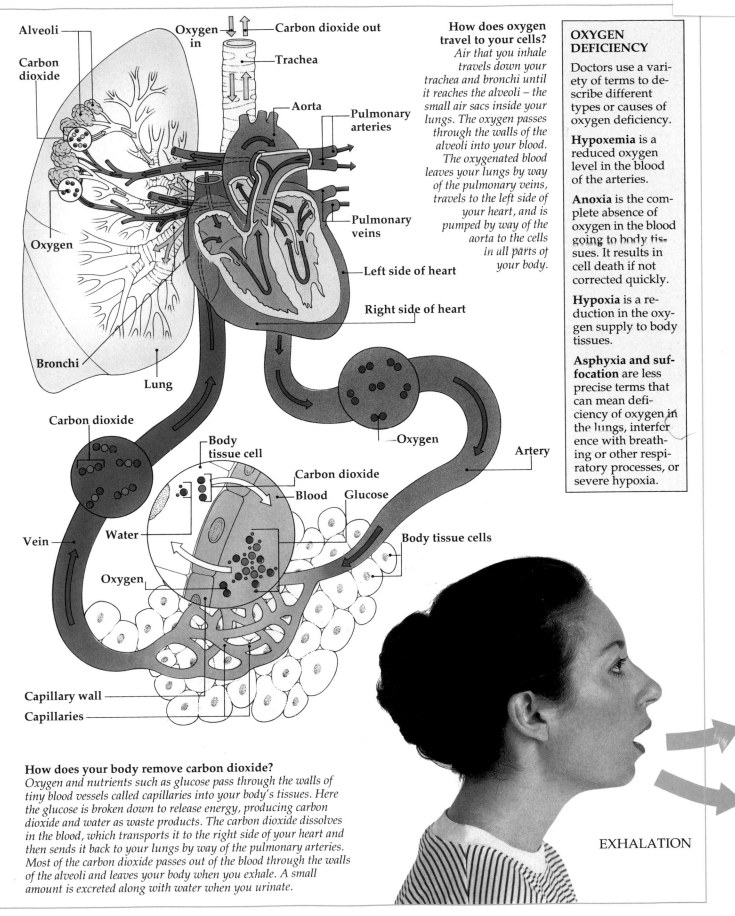

Alveoli

Carbon dioxide

Oxygen in — Carbon dioxide out

Trachea

Aorta

Pulmonary arteries

Pulmonary veins

Left side of heart

Right side of heart

Oxygen

Bronchi

Lung

Carbon dioxide

Body tissue cell

Carbon dioxide

Blood

Glucose

Oxygen

Body tissue cells

Artery

Vein

Water

Oxygen

Capillary wall

Capillaries

How does oxygen travel to your cells?
Air that you inhale travels down your trachea and bronchi until it reaches the alveoli – the small air sacs inside your lungs. The oxygen passes through the walls of the alveoli into your blood. The oxygenated blood leaves your lungs by way of the pulmonary veins, travels to the left side of your heart, and is pumped by way of the aorta to the cells in all parts of your body.

OXYGEN DEFICIENCY

Doctors use a variety of terms to describe different types or causes of oxygen deficiency.

Hypoxemia is a reduced oxygen level in the blood of the arteries.

Anoxia is the complete absence of oxygen in the blood going to body tissues. It results in cell death if not corrected quickly.

Hypoxia is a reduction in the oxygen supply to body tissues.

Asphyxia and suffocation are less precise terms that can mean deficiency of oxygen in the lungs, interference with breathing or other respiratory processes, or severe hypoxia.

How does your body remove carbon dioxide?
Oxygen and nutrients such as glucose pass through the walls of tiny blood vessels called capillaries into your body's tissues. Here the glucose is broken down to release energy, producing carbon dioxide and water as waste products. The carbon dioxide dissolves in the blood, which transports it to the right side of your heart and then sends it back to your lungs by way of the pulmonary arteries. Most of the carbon dioxide passes out of the blood through the walls of the alveoli and leaves your body when you exhale. A small amount is excreted along with water when you urinate.

EXHALATION

11

HOW DO OTHER ANIMALS BREATHE?

All animals – mammals, birds, fish, insects, and amphibians – need oxygen to survive. Some animals have lungs like ours, but others, such as insects and fish, use different methods to extract oxygen from the air or water in which they live.

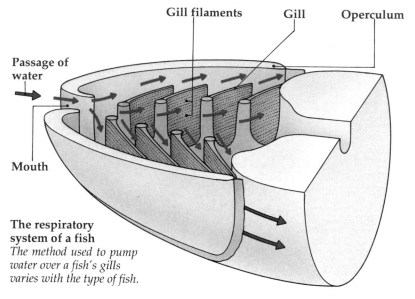

Gill filaments   **Gill**   **Operculum**

Passage of water

Mouth

The respiratory system of a fish
The method used to pump water over a fish's gills varies with the type of fish.

FISH

A fish takes water in through its mouth. The water travels over its gills, which absorb oxygen from the water and pass the oxygen into the fish's blood through thin gill filaments. The water then travels through the operculum, a bony covering over the gills, back to the outside. Although air contains more oxygen than water does, a fish taken out of water will suffocate, because its gill filaments stick together, reducing its intake of oxygen; its muscular system, which includes its mouth, stops functioning. A fish does not use its nostrils to breathe air. The nostrils connect to sensitive organs that detect the presence of food chemicals in water.

ARACHNIDS

Some arachnids, such as scorpions and spiders, breathe through respiratory organs called book lungs. These organs lie in the front of the arachnid's abdomen in a cavity that has a narrow opening to the outside. A number of thin, hollow plates, arranged like the pages of a book, project from the inside wall of the cavity. Blood circulates through the book "pages," taking in oxygen from the air and releasing carbon dioxide.

A spider's book lung
The "pages" of the book lung lie in a depression in the body wall.

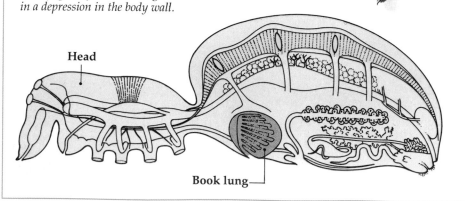

Head

Book lung

The scorpion's book lungs
Like the spider, the scorpion breathes through book lungs. As blood circulates in the shelflike plates, oxygen from the air passes into the blood, and carbon dioxide passes out.

FROGS

The skin of a frog enables it to breathe both in and out of water. A frog's skin is moist, thin, and richly supplied with blood vessels that branch into capillaries. Oxygen from air and water dissolves on the frog's moist skin and passes into the frog's blood. The waste product carbon dioxide also passes out through its skin. When a frog is inactive, breathing through its skin fulfills its energy needs. But when the frog is active and out of the water, it must gulp extra air into its lungs through its mouth.

A frog's versatile lungs
A frog can inflate its lungs to many times their usual size. This ability helps the frog breathe and frightens away predators.

INSECTS

An insect's body contains air tubes (much like your trachea) that open up to the outside through pores (spiracles). The air tubes branch into smaller tubes that allow oxygen to pass directly into every part of the insect's body. Most carbon dioxide travels back out through the air tubes. The rest passes out through the insect's body.

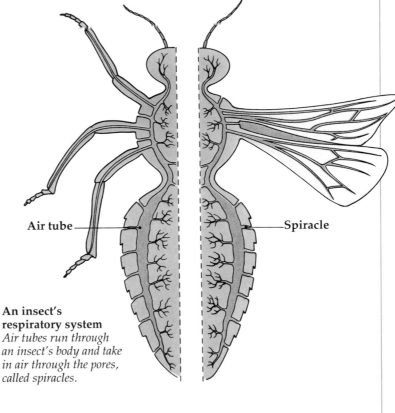

Air tube — — Spiracle

An insect's respiratory system
Air tubes run through an insect's body and take in air through the pores, called spiracles.

BIRDS

Eight or nine air sacs occupy much of the body cavity of a bird. The sacs connect to the bird's lungs. When the bird inhales, air flows into the rear air sacs, while air already in the lungs flows into the front air sacs. As the bird exhales, air flows from the rear sacs into the lungs and air in the front sacs is expelled to the outside. In the lungs, the air passes through small tubes called parabronchi (not shown). Numerous small pockets in the walls of the parabronchi absorb oxygen into the blood. This highly efficient system allows birds to breathe easily while flying at high altitudes where the air oxygen content is low.

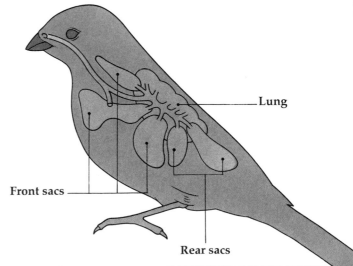

— Lung

Front sacs —

Rear sacs

THE BREATHING PLANET

The Earth's atmosphere contains about 21 percent oxygen. But shortly after the Earth was formed, there was virtually no oxygen free (unbound to other elements) in the atmosphere. Respiration was impossible. The earliest life-forms relied on less efficient processes to obtain energy from simple compounds present in the primitive oceans.

As life evolved, organisms we now call plants developed. They could use sunlight to make and store energy-containing carbohydrates from water and carbon dioxide in the atmosphere. This process is called photosynthesis. As a byproduct of photosynthesis, free oxygen molecules were released – in the oceans and in the atmosphere.

Solar energy

Origins of respiration

As oxygen built up in the atmosphere, more advanced life-forms were able to evolve that had the ability to respire. Eventually, respiration became the dominant method by which organisms produced energy. At the same time, some of the oxygen in the atmosphere formed into ozone, a gas that effectively screens the Earth from harmful high-energy radiation from the sun. The progressive increase in the amount of oxygen in the atmosphere and the formation of the ozone shield were probably the major factors that permitted life to leave the oceans and move onto land.

OXYGEN EQUILIBRIUM

All forms of animal life on the planet, including human life, are highly dependent on plants, which release oxygen. Plants, in turn, need the carbon dioxide that animals exhale to make carbohydrates.

Photosynthesis
Using the pigment chlorophyll, plants capture the energy in sunlight and use it to convert carbon dioxide in the atmosphere into carbohydrates and other substances needed for growth and storage of energy. This process, called photosynthesis, also requires water. Photosynthesis releases oxygen into the atmosphere.

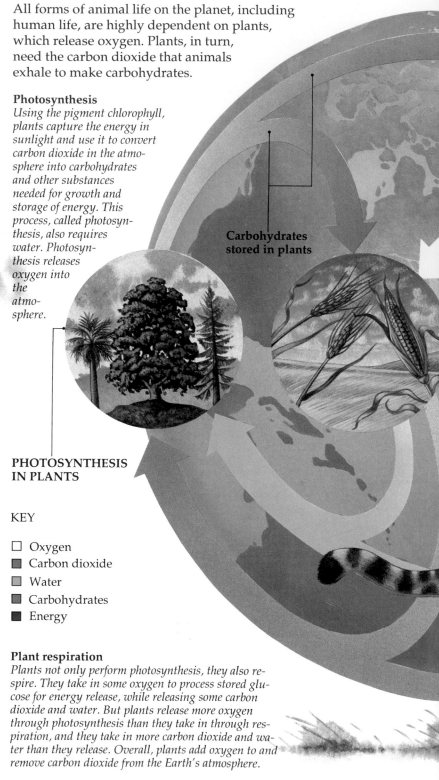

Carbohydrates stored in plants

PHOTOSYNTHESIS IN PLANTS

KEY

☐ Oxygen
■ Carbon dioxide
■ Water
■ Carbohydrates
■ Energy

Plant respiration
Plants not only perform photosynthesis, they also respire. They take in some oxygen to process stored glucose for energy release, while releasing some carbon dioxide and water. But plants release more oxygen through photosynthesis than they take in through respiration, and they take in more carbon dioxide and water than they release. Overall, plants add oxygen to and remove carbon dioxide from the Earth's atmosphere.

Animal respiration

All forms of animal life, including humans, take in oxygen and use it to break down energy-containing substances, principally glucose, to release energy. Carbon dioxide and water are formed as by-products. Animals obtain the energy-containing substances they need, such as glucose, from the food they eat. Ultimately, all food energy comes from the carbohydrates made by photosynthesizing plants. So animal life depends on plant life for both oxygen and food energy.

RESPIRATION BY ANIMALS

Glucose from food

RESPIRATION BY PLANTS

Energy used by animals

GLOBAL WARMING

The level of carbon dioxide in the atmosphere is rising, partly because of the burning of fuels, such as oil and coal, and partly because of the destruction of forests. The loss of trees reduces the planet's capacity to remove carbon dioxide from the air. Rising carbon dioxide levels cause global warming, which is a rise in the temperature of the Earth's atmosphere and oceans, because of the greenhouse effect (see below). Increased carbon dioxide levels have not yet reduced atmospheric oxygen levels much. But global warming could increase the Earth's average temperature dramatically in the future.

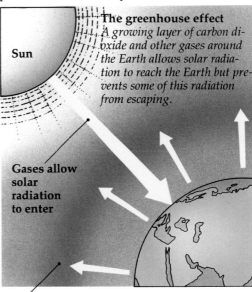

Sun

The greenhouse effect
A growing layer of carbon dioxide and other gases around the Earth allows solar radiation to reach the Earth but prevents some of this radiation from escaping.

Gases allow solar radiation to enter

Layer of carbon dioxide and other gases prevents some radiation from leaving

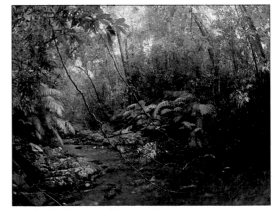

Rain forest destruction
About half of all rain forests have been destroyed. This destruction has diminished the Earth's ability to remove carbon dioxide from the atmosphere.

YOUR RESPIRATORY TRACT

Air enters and leaves your body through your nose or mouth and travels to and from your lungs via your respiratory tract. When you breathe through your nose, air is filtered before it enters your lungs.

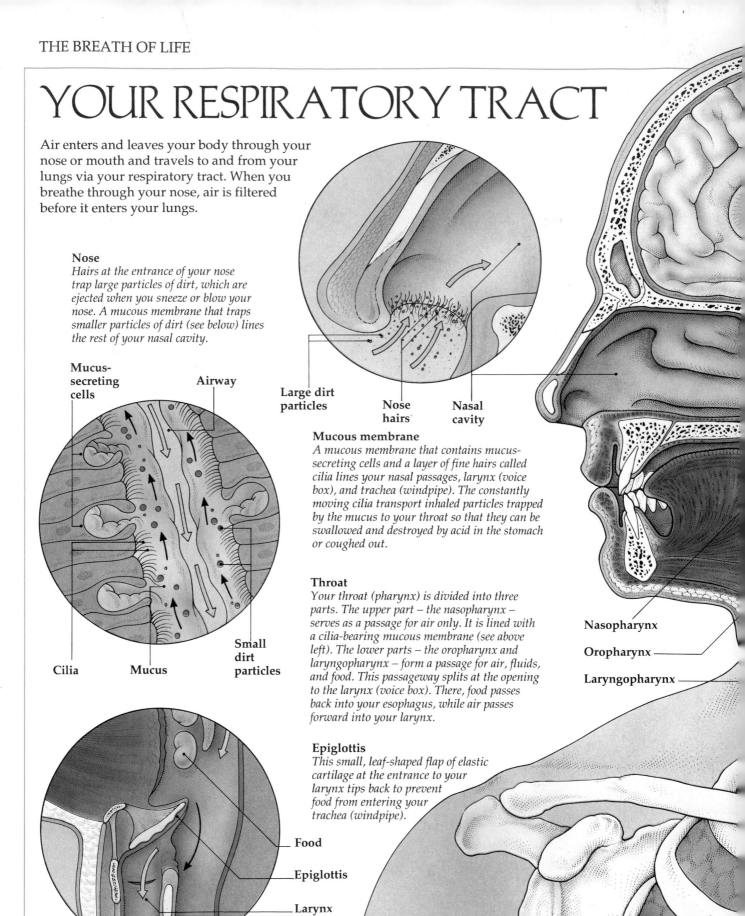

Nose
Hairs at the entrance of your nose trap large particles of dirt, which are ejected when you sneeze or blow your nose. A mucous membrane that traps smaller particles of dirt (see below) lines the rest of your nasal cavity.

Mucus-secreting cells

Airway

Cilia

Mucus

Small dirt particles

Large dirt particles

Nose hairs

Nasal cavity

Mucous membrane
A mucous membrane that contains mucus-secreting cells and a layer of fine hairs called cilia lines your nasal passages, larynx (voice box), and trachea (windpipe). The constantly moving cilia transport inhaled particles trapped by the mucus to your throat so that they can be swallowed and destroyed by acid in the stomach or coughed out.

Throat
Your throat (pharynx) is divided into three parts. The upper part – the nasopharynx – serves as a passage for air only. It is lined with a cilia-bearing mucous membrane (see above left). The lower parts – the oropharynx and laryngopharynx – form a passage for air, fluids, and food. This passageway splits at the opening to the larynx (voice box). There, food passes back into your esophagus, while air passes forward into your larynx.

Nasopharynx

Oropharynx

Laryngopharynx

Epiglottis
This small, leaf-shaped flap of elastic cartilage at the entrance to your larynx tips back to prevent food from entering your trachea (windpipe).

Food

Epiglottis

Larynx

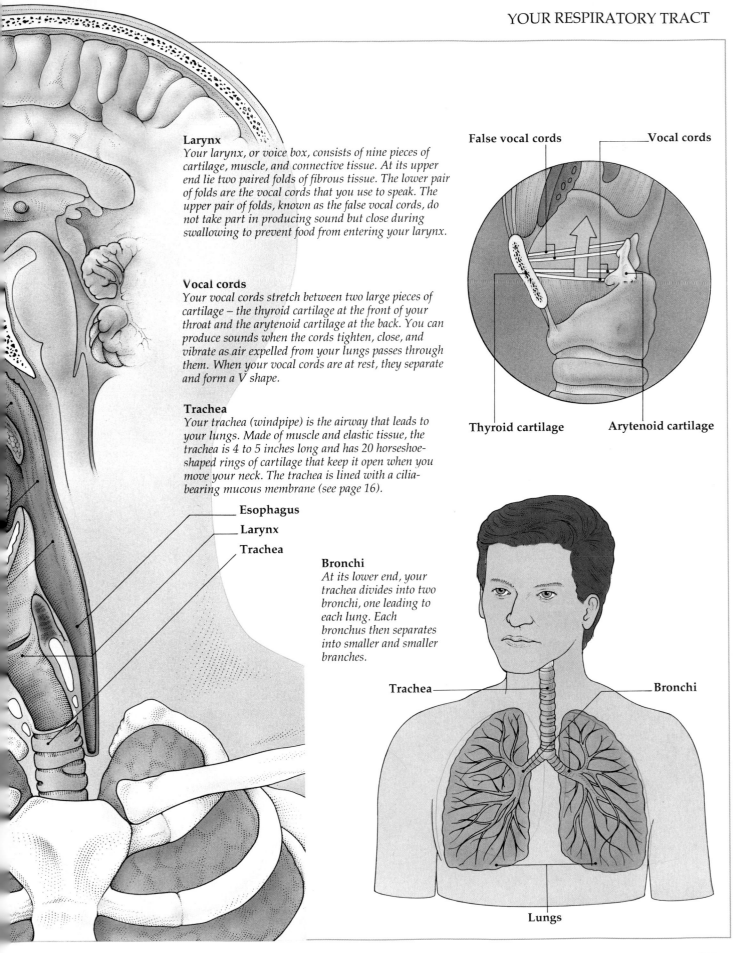

Larynx

Your larynx, or voice box, consists of nine pieces of cartilage, muscle, and connective tissue. At its upper end lie two paired folds of fibrous tissue. The lower pair of folds are the vocal cords that you use to speak. The upper pair of folds, known as the false vocal cords, do not take part in producing sound but close during swallowing to prevent food from entering your larynx.

Vocal cords

Your vocal cords stretch between two large pieces of cartilage – the thyroid cartilage at the front of your throat and the arytenoid cartilage at the back. You can produce sounds when the cords tighten, close, and vibrate as air expelled from your lungs passes through them. When your vocal cords are at rest, they separate and form a V shape.

Trachea

Your trachea (windpipe) is the airway that leads to your lungs. Made of muscle and elastic tissue, the trachea is 4 to 5 inches long and has 20 horseshoe-shaped rings of cartilage that keep it open when you move your neck. The trachea is lined with a cilia-bearing mucous membrane (see page 16).

False vocal cords

Vocal cords

Thyroid cartilage

Arytenoid cartilage

Esophagus

Larynx

Trachea

Bronchi

At its lower end, your trachea divides into two bronchi, one leading to each lung. Each bronchus then separates into smaller and smaller branches.

Trachea

Bronchi

Lungs

17

YOUR LUNGS

Your lungs are two cone-shaped organs that lie on either side of the central cavity in your chest, called the mediastinum. The lungs consist of spongelike tissue made up of thousands of tiny air sacs, called alveoli. This tissue fills the spaces between a branching, treelike network of air tubes and blood vessels in the lungs (see THE BRONCHIAL TREE on page 20). The bottom surfaces of your lungs rest on your diaphragm, a sheet of muscle that arches up into your chest cavity, completely separating it from your abdomen. The upper tips of your lungs extend into your neck, about an inch and a half above the level of your collarbones. The lungs lie within your rib cage.

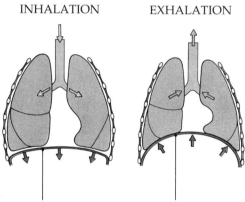

INHALATION   EXHALATION

Contracted diaphragm   Relaxed diaphragm

STRUCTURE OF THE LUNGS

Trachea
The main airway to your lungs – the trachea – divides into two main tubes (bronchi). One bronchus extends into your right lung and the other into your left lung.

Main bronchi – right and left

Right lung
Your right lung has three lobes – the upper, middle, and lower lobes. Each lobe is supplied by a branch of a main bronchus; these branches are called main stem bronchi. The lobes subdivide into segments, each supplied by a segmental bronchus.

Diaphragm
This sheet of muscle separates your chest cavity from your abdominal cavity. When contracted during inhalation, your diaphragm moves downward, allowing your lungs to fill with air. When relaxed during exhalation, it arches upward, helping you to expel air.

Upper lobe

Middle lobe

Lower lobe

Diaphragm

DEVELOPMENT OF LUNGS IN AN EMBRYO

Billions of years ago, organisms that lived in water gradually evolved into creatures that adapted to an environment on land. They began to breathe air. A developing human embryo mimics human evolution. The consecutive stages of the embryo's developing respiratory system resemble the respiratory systems found in fish, amphibians, reptiles, and lower mammals.

A developing human embryo
A bud grows from the tube that will become the embryo's stomach and forms a new tube. The upper part of the new tube develops into the larynx (voice box), and the middle part develops into the trachea (windpipe). The lower part divides into two branches, the lung buds, which later develop into the bronchi and the lung tissue.

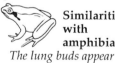 **Similarities with amphibians**
The lung buds appear in a human embryo at 4 to 5 weeks. This stage of development resembles the respiratory system of amphibians, in which the lungs consist of two air sacs.

Stomach tube

Area that will become the larynx

Lung buds

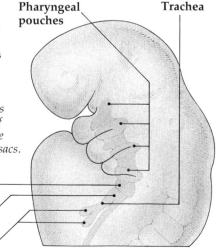

Pharyngeal pouches   Trachea

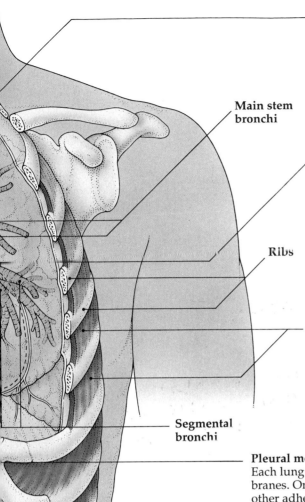

Left lung
Your left lung has two lobes – the upper lobe and the lower lobe. Each is supplied by a main stem bronchus. The lobes further subdivide into segments. Each of these is supplied by a segmental bronchus.

Hilus
The hilus is a depression on the mediastinal (inner) surface of your lungs into which several structures enter – blood vessels connect the lungs to your heart, the main bronchi connect the lungs to your trachea, and connective tissue holds these junctures in place.

Mediastinum
This is the middle part of your chest cavity, located between your lungs. It contains many of the organs in your chest, such as the heart, major blood vessels, esophagus, nerves, and associated connective tissue.

Rib cage
Your rib cage surrounds your chest cavity. It consists of 12 pairs of ribs, the breastbone (sternum), and the flexible cartilage that joins the ribs to the breastbone. Your rib cage protects the vital organs contained in your chest. The intercostal muscles between the ribs and the diaphragm under your lungs rhythmically alter the volume of your rib cage as you breathe.

Main stem bronchi

Ribs

Segmental bronchi

Intercostal muscles
Located between the ribs, the intercostal muscles work together to allow your rib cage to expand and contract during breathing.

Pleural membranes
Each lung is enclosed by two pleural membranes. One adheres firmly to the lung and the other adheres to the inside of the chest wall and to the sides of the mediastinum. Between these two layers lies a thin film of lubricating fluid, called the pleural fluid, that allows the two layers to slide freely against each other as your lungs expand and contract during breathing.

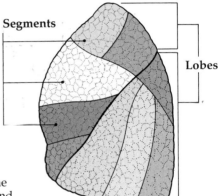

Segments

Lobes

Lobes and segments of the lungs
The colors in the illustration of the left lung (above) show how it is divided into lobes and segments.

Similarities with fish
In humans and land animals, outgrowths called pharyngeal pouches develop into nonrespiratory structures, such as the thyroid glands and the auditory (hearing) tubes. Primitive versions of these structures are present in the 6- to 7-week-old human embryo. In fish, pharyngeal pouches develop into gills.

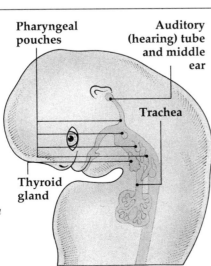

Pharyngeal pouches

Auditory (hearing) tube and middle ear

Trachea

Thyroid gland

Similarities with reptiles
At 7 to 8 weeks, the lungs of the human embryo have developed branching airways (bronchi). At this stage of development they resemble the lungs of reptiles, which have branching respiratory tubes that end in air sacs. Similar air sacs in humans are called alveoli.

Bronchi

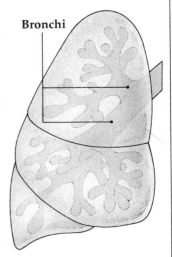

THE BRONCHIAL TREE

The lower respiratory system is made up of your lungs and the airways that begin at your larynx. To ensure that your blood efficiently absorbs the oxygen in the air you breathe, each breath must reach your lung tissue, where oxygen is exchanged for carbon dioxide. The air you inhale travels through an intricate system of successively branching airways that runs throughout the lung tissue. These airways become increasingly narrow until the smallest tubes reach the fragile air sacs from which oxygen passes into your blood. The branching airways resemble an upside down tree – your trachea is the trunk. A similar branching network of blood vessels parallels this bronchial tree. Some blood vessels supply nutrients to the lung's tissues. Others transport blood from your general circulation to and from lung tissue, where the blood absorbs oxygen and releases carbon dioxide.

Smallest airways
Segmental bronchi divide into 50 to 80 terminal bronchioles. Each of these divides into two or more respiratory bronchioles. Finally, each respiratory bronchiole divides into two or more alveolar ducts, which end in air sacs called alveoli.

Terminal bronchiole

Respiratory bronchiole

Capillaries (blood vessels)

Alveoli (air sacs)

Alveolar duct

Main stem bronchi of the right lung
Three main stem bronchi branch from the right main bronchus. They supply the three lobes of the right lung.

Segmental bronchi of the right lung
The three main stem bronchi of the right lung divide into 10 segmental bronchi. They supply the right lung's 10 segments.

Trachea
The trachea (windpipe) is a tube composed of smooth muscle, elastic connective tissue, and fibrous cartilage tissue. Its upper end is connected to the larynx (voice box). Its lower end divides into the two main airways to the lungs – the right and left main bronchi.

Main bronchi
The two main bronchi are composed of material similar to the trachea. The right one supplies the right lung; the left one supplies the left lung. The right main bronchus is shorter and more vertical than the left so that if a small object is inhaled, it usually ends up in the right lung.

Segmental bronchus

Fragile air spaces of the lungs
Alveoli are tiny, elastic sacs. Air that you inhale enters the alveoli through the smallest bronchioles. Minute blood vessels called capillaries bring blood close to the walls of the alveoli, where oxygen is exchanged for carbon dioxide. The oxygen-rich blood then returns to the heart.

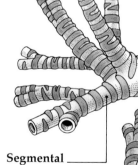

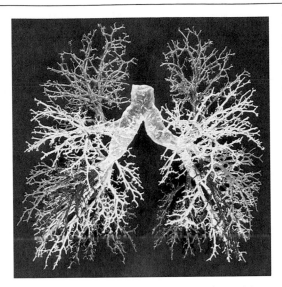

Branching tree
In the photograph at left, a cast of the human airways shows the intricate branching of the bronchial tree. The different colors represent the segmented branches of the bronchi.

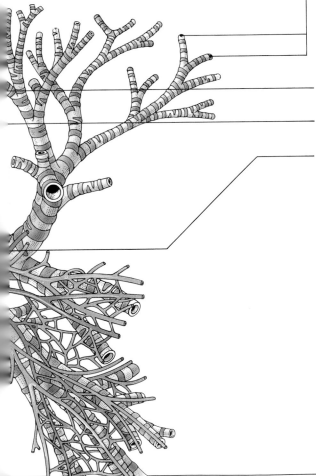

Main stem bronchi of the left lung
Two main stem bronchi branch from the left main bronchus. They supply the lobes of the left lung.

Segmental bronchi of the left lung
The two main stem bronchi of the left lung divide into segmental bronchi. They supply the segments of the left lung.

Bronchioles
Many tiny airways, called bronchioles, branch from the segmental bronchi. Bronchioles end in clusters of air sacs, called alveoli, deep inside the lungs.

Bronchial artery

Bronchial vein

Main stem bronchus

Network of blood vessels
Branching arteries and veins parallel the bronchial tree. The pulmonary (lung-related) circulation carries blood to and from the air sacs, called alveoli, where oxygen enters the blood and carbon dioxide is released. Other blood vessels called bronchial arteries and veins provide the airways and lung tissues with nutrients.

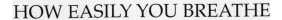

HOW EASILY YOU BREATHE

Two factors play a role in determining the ease with which you breathe. One factor, compliance, is the ability of your lungs and chest to increase in volume. The greater the compliance, the less work it takes to expand your chest and lungs.

Compliance – or elasticity – depends on the ability of your lungs to stretch and then return to their original size. Lung elasticity is determined by several parts of the respiratory system, including a lubricating substance called surfactant (see page 28), which makes inflating the alveoli easier and reduces their tendency to collapse.

The other factor, resistance, refers to how easily air flows into and out of your lungs. The greater the resistance, the more work it takes to inhale and exhale. Resistance depends on the diameter of your airways and their freedom from obstruction by mucus or fluid.

Effects of lung diseases

Increased airway resistance is a more common cause of breathing difficulty than reduced compliance. For example, in a person with asthma, mucus buildup and airway constriction interfere with the flow of air. The person must work hard to move air in and out. Together, compliance and resistance determine how much energy you use to breathe. A person at rest expends about 5 percent of his or her energy output on breathing. If a person has a lung-related disease that reduces compliance or increases resistance, the amount of energy he or she expends on breathing may be as high as 30 percent of energy output. Compliance is reduced by a disease such as pulmonary fibrosis, in which scar tissue replaces normal lung tissue. Resistance is increased by a disease such as asthma, in which airways become obstructed by mucus or fluid. If any of these diseases becomes severe, the respiratory muscles can fail and the person can die.

LUNGS AND CIRCULATION

The blood in your body travels through two sets of circuits – the systemic (total body) circulation and the pulmonary (lung-related) circulation. In the systemic circulation, oxygen-rich blood entering the left side of your heart is pumped throughout your body to supply your cells with oxygen and other nutrients. The blood returns to the right side of the heart after releasing much of its oxygen and acquiring carbon dioxide. From there, the oxygen-deficient blood is pumped through the pulmonary circulation to the lungs. There the blood is replenished with oxygen from the air you breathe, and carbon dioxide is released so you can exhale it. The oxygen-rich blood completes its circuit by returning to the left side of the heart.

SYSTEMIC CIRCULATION

1 Oxygen-rich blood moves from the left atrium into the left ventricle of your heart, which pumps it through the aorta (a major artery) and throughout your body to deliver oxygen to your cells.

2 Tiny blood vessels called capillaries come into close contact with your body's cells. They deliver oxygen to the cells and carry away carbon dioxide.

3 Blood returns from the capillaries to the right atrium of the heart via increasingly larger veins that converge to form the venae cavae (the major veins). The blood has lost much of its oxygen and has acquired carbon dioxide from the cells.

4 This oxygen-deficient blood enters the right ventricle of your heart. From there the blood can be pumped to your lungs.

PULMONARY CIRCULATION

1 The right ventricle of your heart pumps oxygen-deficient blood through the pulmonary arteries to both of your lungs.

2 The blood flows through progressively smaller blood vessels to tiny vessels called capillaries. These vessels come in close contact with the alveoli of the lungs.

3 At the alveoli, blood releases much of its carbon dioxide and takes up oxygen from the alveoli. Oxygen-rich blood then travels away from the capillaries of the lungs through increasingly larger vessels that converge to form the pulmonary veins.

4 Oxygen-rich blood then enters the left atrium of your heart, flows into the heart's left ventricle, and is again ready to be pumped throughout your body.

Capillaries

To upper parts of body

Pulmonary arteries
The pulmonary arteries are the only arteries in your body that contain oxygen-deficient blood.

Oxygen-deficient blood

Capillaries of the lungs

Aorta

Pulmonary veins
The pulmonary veins are the only veins in your body that contain oxygen-rich blood. The systemic veins contain oxygen-deficient blood.

Oxygen-rich blood

Venae cavae

Right atrium

Right ventricle

Left atrium

Left ventricle
More power is needed to pump blood throughout the large, systemic circulation, so the left ventricle of your heart has thicker, more muscular walls than the right ventricle.

To lower parts of body

Oxygen-deficient blood

Capillaries

CIRCULATION IN THE FETUS

A fetus does not breathe air. It gets its oxygen and nutrients from its mother's blood by way of the placenta, the organ that links the blood supplies of the mother and fetus. The blood circulation in a fetus differs greatly from that in a baby after birth. In a fetus, only about 12 percent of the blood pumped by the heart flows through the lungs. After birth, all the baby's blood must pass through the lungs to be reoxygenated and to release carbon dioxide. This process requires that a number of changes occur at birth.

BEFORE BIRTH

1 Oxygenated blood passes via the placenta into the umbilical vein, through the ductus venosus, and into the main lower vein to the right atrium of the heart. Blood returning from the upper parts of the body also enters the right atrium.

2 Oxygenated blood entering the right atrium from the main lower vein passes to the left atrium through an opening (the foramen ovale) in the fetus's heart. Most of the blood travels to the fetus's head and upper limbs by way of the aorta (a major artery).

3 Blood entering the right atrium from the main upper vein passes into the pulmonary artery. Most of this blood bypasses the fetus's lungs by going through the ductus arteriosus, which connects the pulmonary artery to the aorta.

4 Some of this blood reaches the lower parts of the fetus's body, but most returns, via the umbilical arteries, to the placenta, where it mixes with the mother's blood.

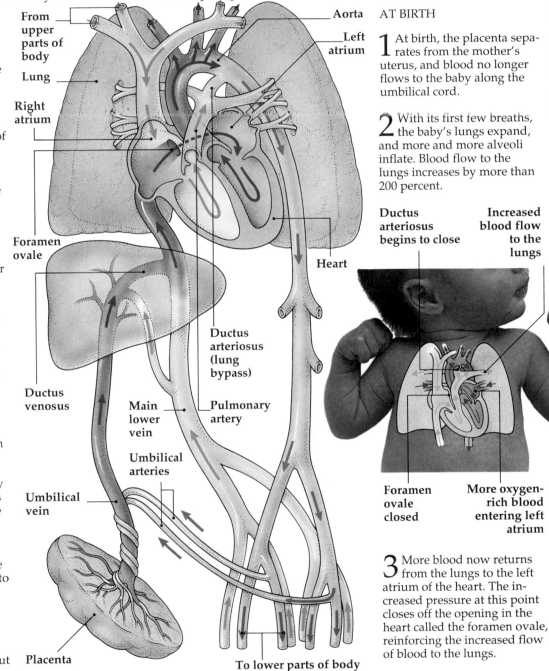

Labels (diagram): From upper parts of body · Lung · Right atrium · Foramen ovale · Ductus venosus · Umbilical vein · Placenta · Aorta · Left atrium · Heart · Ductus arteriosus (lung bypass) · Main lower vein · Pulmonary artery · Umbilical arteries · To lower parts of body · Ductus arteriosus begins to close · Increased blood flow to the lungs · Foramen ovale closed · More oxygen-rich blood entering left atrium

AT BIRTH

1 At birth, the placenta separates from the mother's uterus, and blood no longer flows to the baby along the umbilical cord.

2 With its first few breaths, the baby's lungs expand, and more and more alveoli inflate. Blood flow to the lungs increases by more than 200 percent.

3 More blood now returns from the lungs to the left atrium of the heart. The increased pressure at this point closes off the opening in the heart called the foramen ovale, reinforcing the increased flow of blood to the lungs.

4 The ductus arteriosus (lung bypass) soon closes as the baby's pulmonary vessels increase their capacity to carry blood.

Why are the fetus's lungs bypassed?
In an adult, blood must travel to the lungs to collect oxygen. But a fetus's blood receives oxygen from the mother's blood by way of the placenta. The fluid-filled airways and air sacs inside the fetus's lungs compress the lungs' blood vessels, preventing the flow of blood.

AIR-BLOOD INTERCHANGE

The thin walls of each alveolus lie close to the thin walls of the capillaries in your lungs. At the cellular level, the air in your alveoli and the blood in your capillaries are separated only by a structure called the respiratory membrane, which is made up of the layers located at the point where the alveolar and capillary walls meet (see below). This proximity allows oxygen and carbon dioxide to pass easily between the air in the alveoli and the blood in the capillaries.

Respiratory membrane
The respiratory membrane represents the barrier a molecule of oxygen must cross from the inside of an alveolus to the inside of a capillary. The barrier consists of the fluid layer lining the alveolus, the one-celled alveolar wall, the outer membrane of the alveolus, a fluid-filled space between the alveolus and the capillary, the outer membrane of the capillary, and the capillary cell itself. The structure is only 0.2 thousandth of a millimeter thick.

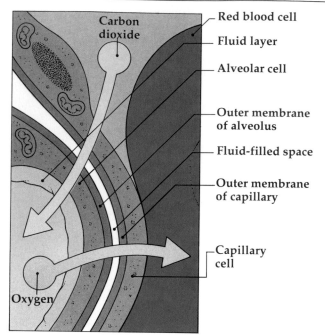

Carbon dioxide

Red blood cell
Fluid layer
Alveolar cell
Outer membrane of alveolus
Fluid-filled space
Outer membrane of capillary
Capillary cell

Oxygen

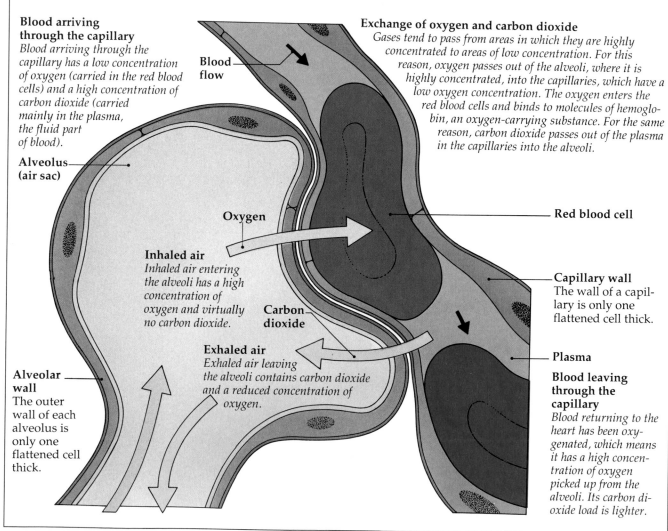

Blood arriving through the capillary
Blood arriving through the capillary has a low concentration of oxygen (carried in the red blood cells) and a high concentration of carbon dioxide (carried mainly in the plasma, the fluid part of blood).

Blood flow

Alveolus (air sac)

Oxygen

Inhaled air
Inhaled air entering the alveoli has a high concentration of oxygen and virtually no carbon dioxide.

Carbon dioxide

Exhaled air
Exhaled air leaving the alveoli contains carbon dioxide and a reduced concentration of oxygen.

Alveolar wall
The outer wall of each alveolus is only one flattened cell thick.

Exchange of oxygen and carbon dioxide
Gases tend to pass from areas in which they are highly concentrated to areas of low concentration. For this reason, oxygen passes out of the alveoli, where it is highly concentrated, into the capillaries, which have a low oxygen concentration. The oxygen enters the red blood cells and binds to molecules of hemoglobin, an oxygen-carrying substance. For the same reason, carbon dioxide passes out of the plasma in the capillaries into the alveoli.

Red blood cell

Capillary wall
The wall of a capillary is only one flattened cell thick.

Plasma

Blood leaving through the capillary
Blood returning to the heart has been oxygenated, which means it has a high concentration of oxygen picked up from the alveoli. Its carbon dioxide load is lighter.

FACTS ABOUT THE LUNGS

A lifetime of breathing

In an average lifetime of 75 years, you will breathe in and out more than 200 million quarts, or 8 million cubic feet, of air. This is enough air to blow up a balloon 125 feet in diameter. It is also enough to have filled the largest dirigible ever built – the Graf Zeppelin V (air capacity 7 million cubic feet).

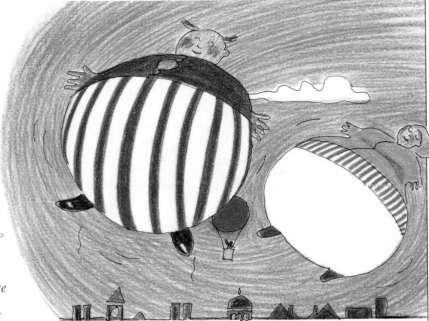

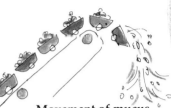

Movement of mucus

The mucous layer lining your respiratory tract is constantly moving toward your mouth – at a rate of about 1 inch per minute – carrying inhaled particles upward to be swallowed or coughed out.

Surface area

In an average-sized adult, the total surface area available for the exchange of oxygen and carbon dioxide in the lungs is about 750 square feet (roughly the size of a regulation badminton court).

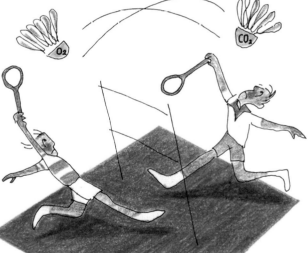
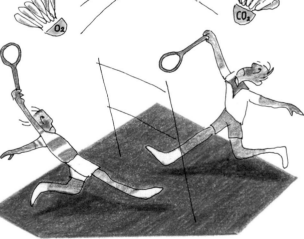

How strong are your lungs?

If you are under water that is more than 9 inches deep, it is impossible to breathe through a pipe that extends to the surface – no matter what you may have seen in the movies. External pressure on your chest increases with depth. In water deeper than 9 inches, the pressure becomes too great for you to expand your chest.

The power of your sneeze or cough

When you sneeze or cough, you clear secretions and particles from your respiratory tract. The force of a sneeze or cough can be amazingly powerful. Particles expelled during a sneeze or cough can travel faster than 100 miles per hour.

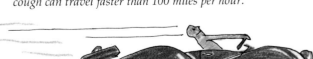

THE LUNG'S DEFENSES

You breathe about 10,000 quarts of air every day. This means that your lungs are exposed to attack by a number of hazards present in the air, such as microorganisms or airborne particles. But your respiratory system has several ways of fighting back, both physical and chemical.

PHYSICAL BARRIERS

The hairs that line your nose can filter out large airborne particles, but not smaller ones that can also be harmful. The specialized lining of the air tubes (see below) protects you from many of these smaller particles.

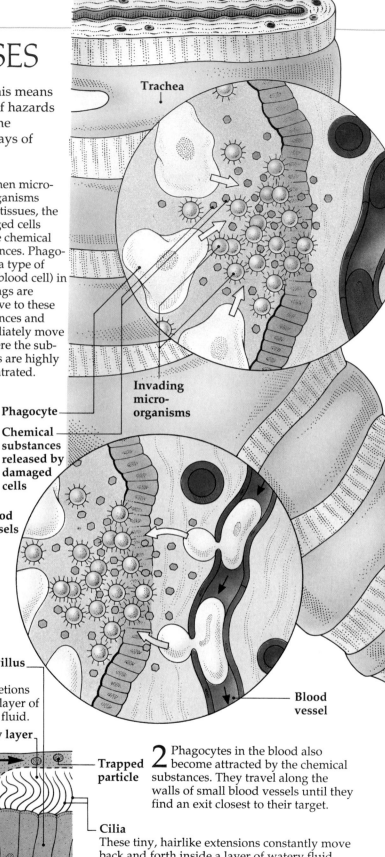

1 When microorganisms attack tissues, the damaged cells release chemical substances. Phagocytes (a type of white blood cell) in the lungs are sensitive to these substances and immediately move to where the substances are highly concentrated.

Trachea

Invading microorganisms

Phagocyte

Chemical substances released by damaged cells

Blood vessels

Blood vessel

A trap for airborne particles
The inner surface of your air tubes is made of a mucous membrane that contains mucus-secreting cells and a layer of cells bearing millions of fine, hairlike extensions called cilia (see the color-enhanced photograph below, magnified 500 times). The cilia move like a wind-blown field to transport particles that have been trapped by the mucus up toward your mouth. When they reach the trachea or major airways, you can expel the particles by coughing. You can also swallow them when they reach the throat.

CROSS SECTION OF TRACHEA

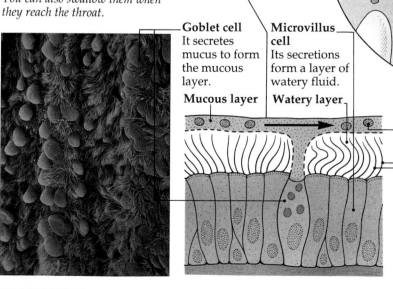

Goblet cell
It secretes mucus to form the mucous layer.

Microvillus cell
Its secretions form a layer of watery fluid.

Mucous layer   **Watery layer**

Trapped particle

2 Phagocytes in the blood also become attracted by the chemical substances. They travel along the walls of small blood vessels until they find an exit closest to their target.

Cilia
These tiny, hairlike extensions constantly move back and forth inside a layer of watery fluid. Their tips project into the mucous layer and move it up toward the trachea. Smoking reduces the motion of the cilia, diminishing your lungs' ability to clear out particles and secretions.

HOW THE IMMUNE SYSTEM FIGHTS INVADERS

Microorganisms, such as bacteria and viruses, that enter the respiratory tract spur your immune system into action. There are millions of white blood cells called phagocytes in the respiratory tract and in the blood. They become attracted to sites of infection where they engulf and destroy invading microorganisms.

3 Proteins, called antibodies, produced by the immune system, help the phagocytes recognize the organisms by attaching themselves to the invaders. Because phagocytes have receptors for the antibodies, the invading organisms attached to the antibodies become stuck to the phagocytes.

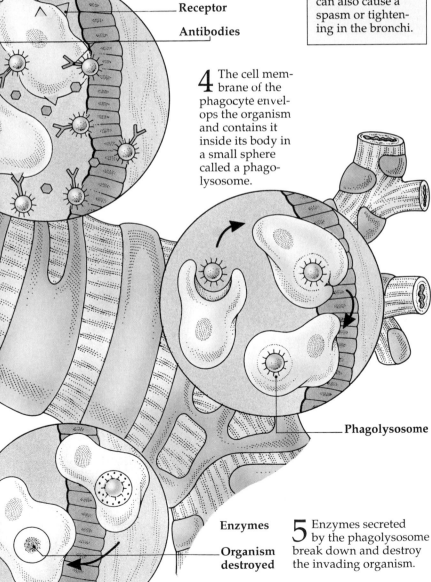

Receptor

Antibodies

4 The cell membrane of the phagocyte envelops the organism and contains it inside its body in a small sphere called a phagolysosome.

Phagolysosome

Enzymes

Organism destroyed

5 Enzymes secreted by the phagolysosome break down and destroy the invading organism.

ALLERGY

Sometimes your immune system perceives a threat in something harmless to most people, such as cat fur. Its reaction is called an allergy. In people who have hay fever, pollen stimulates some white blood cells to release a substance called histamine. This irritating substance produces a stuffy nose and itchy, watery eyes. In people with asthma, histamine can also cause a spasm or tightening in the bronchi.

WHAT HAPPENS WHEN YOU COUGH?

Coughing is a beneficial and protective reflex that clears irritants from your trachea and bronchi. The cough reflex is initiated by messages from receptors in your airways that are sensitive to stimulation by inhaled particles or harmful chemicals, such as automobile exhaust. The messages travel to a center in the brain stem, which triggers the cough.

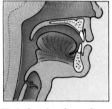 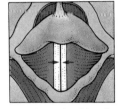

Epiglottis closed   **Vocal cords closed**

1 First, you take a deep breath, your epiglottis closes, and your vocal cords press together to trap air in your lungs.

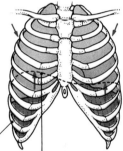

2 Your lungs are compressed by your rising diaphragm and the contraction of the muscles in your abdomen, between your ribs, and in your chest wall.

Rib cage   **Diaphragm**

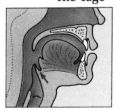 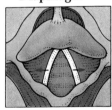

Epiglottis open   **Vocal cords open**

3 When the pressure is at its maximum, your vocal cords suddenly separate and your epiglottis opens.

4 A blast of air passes up your airway and out through your mouth, carrying inhaled particles with it.

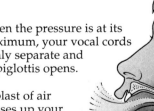

**Alcohol on
your breath**
*Although only a small
proportion of the alcohol
a person drinks is
exhaled, a product of the
metabolism of alcohol in
the body, called acetalde-
hyde, leaves a detectable
odor on the drinker's
breath for several hours
after drinking.*

**HELP FOR
PREMATURE
BABIES**

During the last
decade, research
conducted on
hundreds of
newborns has led
to a lifesaving
treatment for
premature babies.
Very premature
infants who are not
born with enough
surfactant (see
right) to breathe
normally can be
given a form of
surfactant derived
from cows. Within
15 minutes after
birth, the substance
is introduced into
the baby's lungs
through a tube
inserted into the
trachea (windpipe).
Studies show that
the treatment
reduces deaths
from newborn
respiratory distress
syndrome by at
least 55 percent.

EVAPORATION OF FLUID
FROM YOUR LUNGS

The membranes that line your airways contain many glands and
cells that secrete fluid to keep
your entire respiratory tract
moist. When you breathe, a
large amount of this fluid is
lost. The rate of water loss depends on
the temperature and the humidity of the
inhaled air and on how fast and how
deeply you breathe. In mild weather
conditions, water loss from breathing
averages about 11 ounces per day. Your
body maintains the total amount of water in your body tissues at a relatively
constant level by causing you to feel
thirsty or have the urge to urinate.

The evaporation of water from your
respiratory tract also causes the loss of a
large amount of heat energy – about
250 calories per day.

Evaporation of
alcohol from the lungs
If you have been drinking alcohol, only a
small amount in your blood passes into
the alveoli in your lungs, evaporates from
the respiratory tract, and leaves your
body when you exhale. Blood levels of
alcohol fall mainly because of the
breakdown of alcohol by your liver.

SURFACTANT: A VITAL SUBSTANCE IN YOUR AIR SACS

One factor that allows your lungs to inflate easily and remain partially inflated
when you exhale is the presence of a substance called surfactant. Surfactant is a
detergentlike liquid that is secreted inside the alveoli, the delicate air sacs inside
your lungs. If your lungs didn't contain surfactant, they would tend to collapse
and it would be virtually impossible for you to breathe. Babies who are born
prematurely sometimes have insufficient amounts of surfactant and develop
newborn respiratory distress syndrome (see page 29).

Forces that cause the alveoli to collapse
*Each alveolus is lined on the inside with a thin layer
of fluid. The molecules of fluid are strongly attracted
both to each other and to the alveolar walls. These
strong forces of attraction tend to pull the walls of
the alveolus inward and cause it to collapse.*

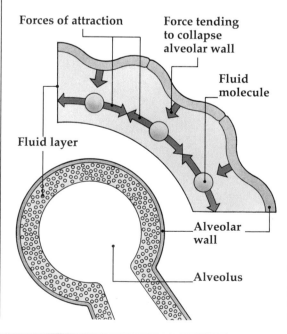

Forces of attraction

Force tending
to collapse
alveolar wall

Fluid
molecule

Fluid layer

Alveolar
wall

Alveolus

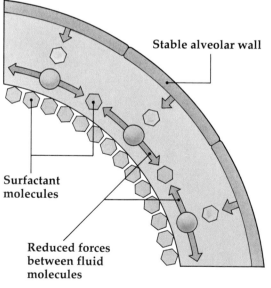

Stable alveolar wall

Surfactant
molecules

Reduced forces
between fluid
molecules

Essential role of surfactant
*Some of the alveolar cells secrete surfactant, which
forms a thin layer over the surface of the fluid layer.
The surfactant molecules intersperse between the
fluid molecules and reduce the forces of attraction
between them. As a result, the alveoli in your lungs
stay inflated and do not collapse.*

SURFACTANT IN THE NEWBORN

The alveoli of a fetus begin to produce surfactant at about the 23rd week of development. But quantities of surfactant sufficient to prevent the alveoli from collapsing when the newborn baby breathes air are produced between the 28th and 32nd weeks of development. A baby born before this time will have diffi culty breathing because of an inadequate supply of surfactant.

Role of surfactant at birth
When a baby takes its first breath, he or she makes a huge physical effort to inflate the fluid-filled airways and alveoli. When the alveoli fill with air for the first time, the surfactant present allows the alveoli to remain partially inflated when the baby exhales. Subsequent breaths become progressively easier as the alveoli inflate more and then remain inflated.

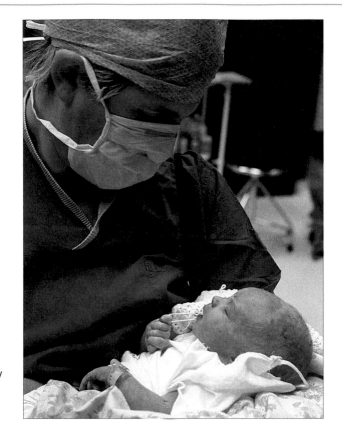

Respiratory distress syndrome
If a baby is born prematurely, surfactant in the alveoli may be reduced or absent. After the baby takes his or her first breath, the alveoli collapse again because of the surfactant deficiency and the baby must exert another huge effort, similar to the first breath, to reinflate them. The baby soon becomes exhausted. Doctors can give the baby inhaled artificial surfactant and mechanical respiration (see page 139).

NORMAL NEWBORN RESPIRATION

NEWBORN RESPIRATORY DISTRESS SYNDROME

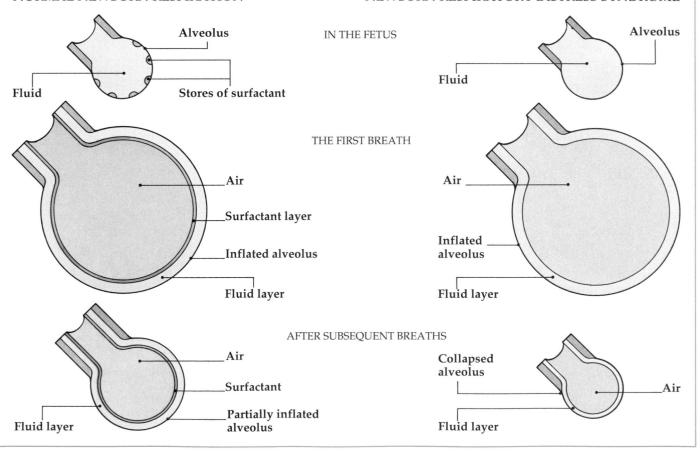

IN THE FETUS

Alveolus

Fluid

Stores of surfactant

Alveolus

Fluid

THE FIRST BREATH

Air

Surfactant layer

Inflated alveolus

Fluid layer

Air

Inflated alveolus

Fluid layer

AFTER SUBSEQUENT BREATHS

Air

Surfactant

Partially inflated alveolus

Fluid layer

Collapsed alveolus

Air

Fluid layer

HOW YOUR BLOOD TRANSPORTS OXYGEN

Once oxygen from your lungs enters your blood, it must be carried efficiently to your body's cells. Your red blood cells and the oxygen-carrying pigment they contain, called hemoglobin, perform this function.

Hemoglobin

Hemoglobin is the substance in red blood cells that carries oxygen to your body's cells. The hemoglobin molecule has two components – heme and globin. Globin is a protein made up of four folded chains of long, stringlike molecules (see below). In normal adult hemoglobin, each folded chain surrounds a molecule of heme, a chemical structure that has an atom of iron at its center.

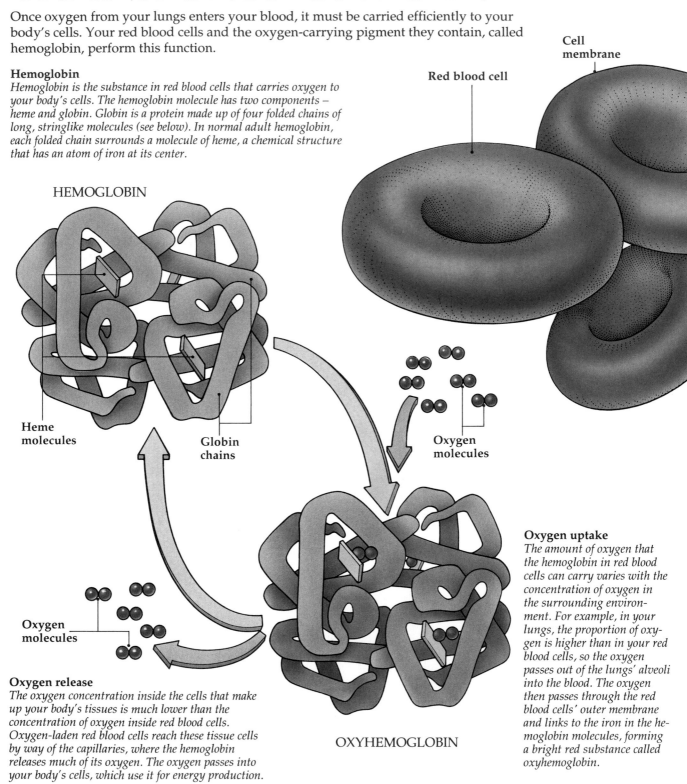

Red blood cell

Cell membrane

HEMOGLOBIN

Heme molecules

Globin chains

Oxygen molecules

Oxygen molecules

OXYHEMOGLOBIN

Oxygen uptake

The amount of oxygen that the hemoglobin in red blood cells can carry varies with the concentration of oxygen in the surrounding environment. For example, in your lungs, the proportion of oxygen is higher than in your red blood cells, so the oxygen passes out of the lungs' alveoli into the blood. The oxygen then passes through the red blood cells' outer membrane and links to the iron in the hemoglobin molecules, forming a bright red substance called oxyhemoglobin.

Oxygen release

The oxygen concentration inside the cells that make up your body's tissues is much lower than the concentration of oxygen inside red blood cells. Oxygen-laden red blood cells reach these tissue cells by way of the capillaries, where the hemoglobin releases much of its oxygen. The oxygen passes into your body's cells, which use it for energy production.

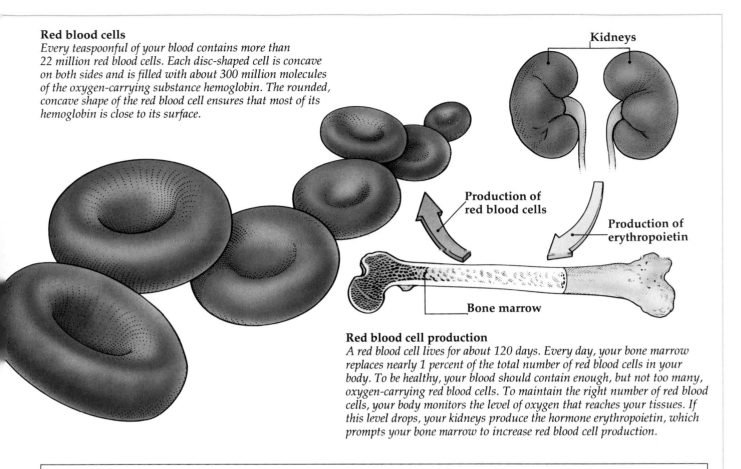

Red blood cells
Every teaspoonful of your blood contains more than 22 million red blood cells. Each disc-shaped cell is concave on both sides and is filled with about 300 million molecules of the oxygen-carrying substance hemoglobin. The rounded, concave shape of the red blood cell ensures that most of its hemoglobin is close to its surface.

Kidneys

Production of red blood cells

Production of erythropoietin

Bone marrow

Red blood cell production
A red blood cell lives for about 120 days. Every day, your bone marrow replaces nearly 1 percent of the total number of red blood cells in your body. To be healthy, your blood should contain enough, but not too many, oxygen-carrying red blood cells. To maintain the right number of red blood cells, your body monitors the level of oxygen that reaches your tissues. If this level drops, your kidneys produce the hormone erythropoietin, which prompts your bone marrow to increase red blood cell production.

HOW ANEMIA AFFECTS THE BLOOD'S ABILITY TO CARRY OXYGEN

When a person has anemia, the amount of hemoglobin circulating in the blood is reduced, either because there are too few red blood cells or because the cells contain too little hemoglobin. This reduction of hemoglobin causes a decrease in the blood's ability to carry oxygen. The red blood cells cannot deliver enough oxygen to the body's cells, which makes the person feel tired and look pale. The body tries to compensate for the oxygen shortage in a number of ways. For example, the heart begins to circulate blood around the body faster, and the cells try to extract more oxygen from the available hemoglobin. But these coping mechanisms do not provide enough oxygen to the cells.

Anemia can be caused by not eating enough iron-containing foods, by menstruation or internal bleeding, or by conditions affecting the bone marrow. Treatment depends on the underlying cause.

Normal red blood cells
The photograph at right (magnified 700 times) shows stained red blood cells in a sample of blood taken from a healthy person. The cells are regular-shaped discs that are concave on each side. They contain the oxygen-carrying pigment hemoglobin, which makes them appear dark red.

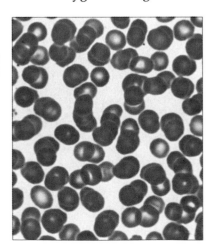

Iron-deficiency anemia
The photograph at right shows stained red blood cells (magnified 360 times) taken from a person with iron-deficiency anemia. The red blood cells appear pale because they contain low amounts of hemoglobin. They are also smaller, misshapen, and fewer in number than healthy red blood cells.

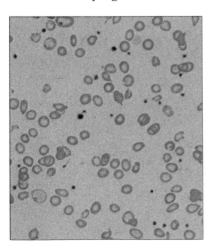

BREATHING

Breathing – the movement of air into and out of your lungs – depends on the differences in pressure between the air outside your body (the atmospheric pressure) and the air inside your lungs. These differences in pressure occur because the volume of your chest cavity changes when your breathing muscles contract and relax.

When you breathe at rest, the volume of your chest cavity changes. Your diaphragm – a muscular sheet that forms the floor of your chest – and your external intercostal muscles, which lie between your ribs, both contract and relax. You use additional muscles in your neck, chest, and abdomen when you breathe in or out forcefully.

HOW DO YOU BREATHE?

HYPER-VENTILATION

Hyperventilation (abnormally deep or rapid, shallow breathing) is especially common during times of anxiety or stress. It causes too much carbon dioxide to be lost from the bloodstream, reducing the acid content of the blood. The person experiences light-headedness, and numbness and tingling in the hands and feet, and around the lips. Someone who is hyperventilating feels as though he or she is not getting enough air, so the person may breathe even faster, which makes the condition worse. Breathing into and out of a paper bag helps reduce the loss of carbon dioxide but should be used only if the person recognizes that the hyperventilation is caused by anxiety, not by a serious disorder.

Before taking a breath
Just before you take a breath, the pressure inside your lungs and the pressure outside your body (atmospheric pressure) are the same. The pressure in the space between the two layers of the pleura, the membrane surrounding the lungs, is just below atmospheric pressure.

As the chest cavity enlarges
Muscle contractions in your diaphragm and between your ribs enlarge the volume of your chest cavity. The resulting drop in the pressure in the pleural space creates a vacuum that causes the lungs to expand. The pressure inside the lungs falls below atmospheric pressure because of their increased volume.

Pleural space

Diaphragm

As you exhale
Your respiratory muscles relax, causing a decrease in the volume of your chest cavity and an increase in pressure inside the pleural space. Your lungs decrease in volume, pressure inside your lungs increases, and air flows out of your mouth until the pressures inside the lungs and in the atmosphere are equal again.

As you inhale
Because air moves from an area of higher pressure to one of lower pressure, air is drawn into your lungs until the pressure inside your lungs is equal to the atmospheric pressure. At this point, the pressure inside the pleural space drops even lower.

BREATHING MUSCLES

— Muscles in the neck

INHALATION

EXHALATION

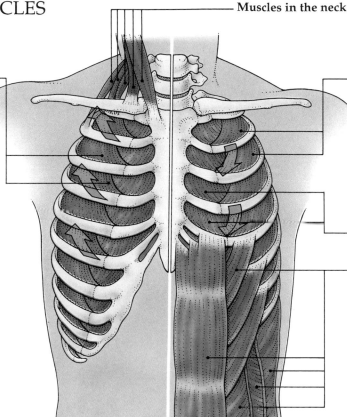

External intercostal muscles
Contraction of these muscles, which lie between the ribs, pulls your ribs together. This causes them to rise and swing outward. These movements increase the horizontal dimension of your chest cavity.

External intercostal muscles
Your rib cage moves downward and inward as the external intercostal muscles between your ribs relax.

— Internal intercostal muscles

— Abdominal muscles

Forceful inhalation
During forceful inhalation – such as during strenuous exercise – you contract the muscles in your neck extending from the base of the skull and the sides of your neck to the inner end of your collarbone and first rib. These contractions increase the horizontal dimension of your chest cavity.

Forceful exhalation
During forceful exhalation, the volume of your chest cavity is decreased even more by the contraction of the internal intercostal muscles (which pull your ribs downward) and of the muscles in your abdomen.

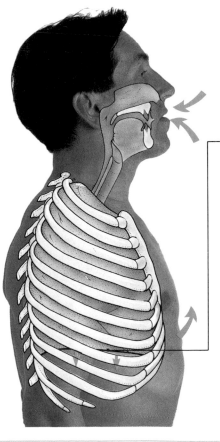

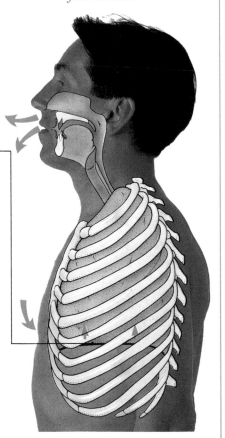

Diaphragm during inhalation
Contracting your diaphragm flattens it, increasing the vertical dimension of your chest cavity.

Diaphragm during exhalation
The diaphragm returns to its relaxed position and elevated, domed shape.

How much air can you breathe?
During a normal inhalation, you take in about a pint of air. But if you breathe in deeply, you can increase this amount by another 5 to 7 pints. During a normal exhalation, you breathe out a pint of air, but you can force another 2 pints out of your lungs. A reserve of air remains in your lungs at any given time. On average, a person breathes in and out about 12 to 17 times per minute while at rest.

WHAT CONTROLS YOUR BREATHING?

Although you can consciously alter its rate and depth, breathing is usually an unconscious process, controlled by nerve centers in the lower part of your brain stem. Various parts of your body send these nerve centers information, by way of your nerves, about the amount of carbon dioxide and oxygen in your blood, your level of physical activity, your emotional state, and the breathing process itself. The nerve centers in your brain stem then adjust your breathing process accordingly.

Respiratory center
Located in the medulla, a part of the brain stem, the respiratory center consists of the inspiratory and the expiratory centers, which control inhaling and exhaling. The respiratory center coordinates the breathing process without your conscious control or awareness.

Inspiratory center
Nerve cells in the inspiratory center send out electrical signals that determine the basic rhythm of breathing. The nerve signals travel down the spinal cord and out along the nerves to the muscles of the rib cage. Nerve signals from the inspiratory center also travel along the nerves attached to both sides of the diaphragm.

Expiratory center
During quiet breathing, nerve cells of the expiratory center are inactive. Exhalation occurs on its own when you relax the muscles in your rib cage and the diaphragm.

Muscles of inhalation
Inhalation is performed mainly by the muscles of the diaphragm and the muscles located between the ribs, called the external intercostal muscles.

Medulla

Chemical sensors in the brain
Located near the medulla, structures called chemoreceptors detect chemical changes in the brain. If the level of carbon dioxide in your blood begins to rise, the chemoreceptors send out nerve signals that stimulate the inspiratory center. The rate and depth of your breathing increases, removing the excess carbon dioxide.

Other breathing stimuli
You begin breathing more rapidly and deeply when you feel pain, experience emotion, or undergo stress, because your body releases hormones such as epinephrine (adrenaline).

Conscious control of breathing
The higher (more recently evolved) centers of your brain allow you to control your breathing to a certain degree, by consciously overriding the nerve centers in the brain stem that control breathing.

Brain stem

Arteries

External intercostal muscles

Internal intercostal muscles

Abdominal muscles

Spinal cord

Nerve signals

Chemical sensors in the arteries
Chemical sensors are also located in some artery walls near your heart and in your neck. If the carbon dioxide levels in your blood increase, these chemical sensors send nerve signals to the inspiratory center to stimulate breathing. Some of these receptors also become activated when the amount of oxygen in your blood falls below a certain critical level.

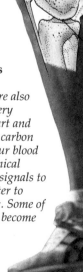

HOW BREATHING CHANGES DURING EXERCISE

When you exercise, your muscles and joints send nerve and chemical signals to your brain, which stimulates the muscles of breathing to increase the rate and depth of the breaths you take. The amount of oxygen in your blood does not decrease during exercise and blood levels of carbon dioxide do not increase. You exhale extra carbon dioxide as rapidly as you produce it.

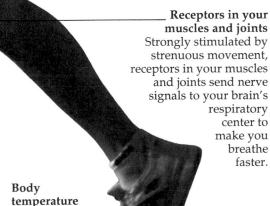

Motor cortex of your brain
The motor cortex of your brain activates the exercising muscles of your body. Nerve signals from the motor cortex stimulate the nerves controlling your chest and diaphragm.

Muscles of the upper part of your chest and shoulders

Airways

Lung

Ribs

Diaphragm

Feedback signals from the lungs
Deep breathing activates structures called stretch receptors in the airways. These receptors send nerve signals to the inspiratory center to limit inhalation and prevent overinflation of your lungs.

Receptors in your muscles and joints
Strongly stimulated by strenuous movement, receptors in your muscles and joints send nerve signals to your brain's respiratory center to make you breathe faster.

Body temperature
A rise in your body temperature, caused by strenuous exercise, also stimulates breathing.

Inspiratory center during exercise
During exercise, nerve cells in your brain's inspiratory center send additional signals to the muscles of the upper part of your chest and shoulders. Your inhalations become greater in volume and more forceful, so air gets into your lungs faster.

Expiratory center during exercise
When you exercise, the expiratory center in your brain sends out nerve signals to activate the muscles of exhalation. You exhale more forcefully, so air gets out of your lungs faster.

Muscles of expiration
The internal intercostal muscles and the abdominal muscles perform forceful exhalation.

Deep breathing
You breathe more deeply during exercise than when you are at rest because deep breathing provides oxygen and disposes of carbon dioxide more efficiently than does rapid, shallower breathing.

TWO TYPES OF EXERCISE

You can perform two types of exercise: aerobic and anaerobic. Aerobic exercise uses oxygen to provide energy for your muscles; anaerobic exercise uses other means (see below). Aerobic activities, such as jogging, improve your endurance and make your heart a more efficient pump. Anaerobic activities, such as weight lifting, make your muscles stronger.

Aerobic exercise
Aerobic exercise is any activity that uses oxygen to provide energy for your muscles. Aerobic exercise uses the large muscles in your trunk, arms, and legs. Forms of aerobic exercise include walking, jogging, biking, and swimming. During aerobic exercise, the rate at which oxygen reaches your muscles equals the rate at which you use up oxygen, so you can sustain the activity for a long time.

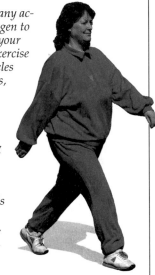

Anaerobic exercise
Weight lifting or sprinting short distances are examples of the short, sharp bursts of activity that characterize anaerobic exercise. Instead of using oxygen, this type of exercise relies on another series of chemical reactions to obtain energy for your muscles. A waste product of this process, lactic acid, accumulates in your muscles, causing them to become fatigued, so you can do anaerobic exercise for only a short time.

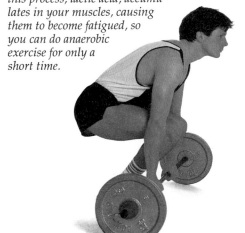

HOLDING YOUR BREATH

If you hold your breath, the rising level of carbon dioxide in your blood quickly stimulates an urge to breathe. If you can withstand this urge, the amount of oxygen reaching your brain eventually falls so low that you could lose consciousness and collapse. Usually, breathing then resumes automatically, under the control of the respiratory center in your brain. You rapidly regain consciousness once the amount of oxygen reaching your brain rises to a normal level.

Breath-holding under water

After years of training, sponge divers and pearl divers can work under water for periods of 5 to 7 minutes without breathing. But most people can hold their breath for only about a minute before they experience an overpowering urge to take another breath.

People who snorkel usually spend part of the time swimming under water holding their breath and part of the time swimming at the surface while breathing through a snorkel, a type of air tube. Snorkeling presents little danger as long as you do not prolong any underwater dive past the point at which you feel an urge to breathe.

Swimmers, divers, and snorkelers should be especially careful not to hyperventilate (breathe abnormally deeply and rapidly) when on the surface of the water. Hyperventilation can be extremely dangerous and is responsible for many water-related deaths. It rapidly releases most of the carbon dioxide from a person's bloodstream (see above right). By the time the person's carbon dioxide level has risen far enough to stimulate breathing, the oxygen level in the person's tissues may have fallen so low that the person could pass out in the water and drown. The most important precaution swimmers, divers, and snorkelers can take is to stay calm and breathe normally while in the water.

SAFE OXYGEN LEVELS FOR A DIVER

A diver without an air tank must breathe calmly immediately before diving. Hyperventilation (breathing abnormally deeply) before diving may suppress the body's urge to breathe. The diver could pass out and drown.

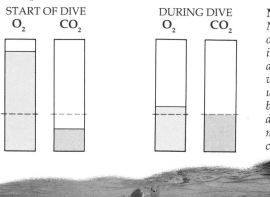

Normal breathing
Normally, the amount of carbon dioxide (CO_2) in the blood during a dive rises to a level at which it stimulates the urge to breathe before blood oxygen (O_2) has dropped below the level needed to maintain consciousness.

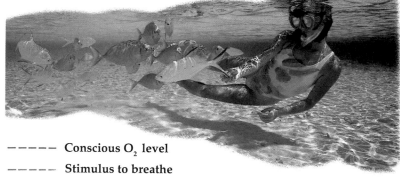

– – – – – **Conscious O_2 level**

– – – – – **Stimulus to breathe**

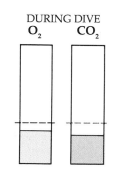

After hyperventilating
Hyperventilation produces a significant fall in the amount of carbon dioxide (CO_2) in the blood. During a dive after hyperventilating, blood oxygen (O_2) may fall below the level required to maintain consciousness before the carbon dioxide level has risen high enough to stimulate breathing.

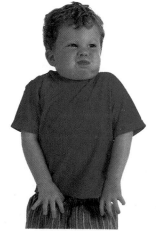

Breath-holding in children
Infants and toddlers may sometimes hold their breath as a response to pain, but they are more often expressing frustration or anger. The child begins to cry and then holds his or her breath. After a few seconds, the child's face turns red or blue. Occasionally, the child faints. When this happens, the body's natural reflexes take over and the child automatically begins to breathe again before any harm is done.

HOW CAN WHALES STAY UNDER WATER SO LONG?

Whales can remain under water longer than any other mammal. To remain under water at such length, the whale's body has become uniquely adapted to its environment. Some large whales remain submerged for 20 minutes or more and can dive thousands of feet. Before they dive, whales do not fill their lungs with air because they would become too buoyant. A large gulp of air would also become compressed at the high water pressures that exist at great depths and much of the air would be dissolved in the whale's blood. If it took a deep breath, dove, and surfaced rapidly, the whale would get "the bends" (see page 39).

Blood circulation changes
A whale's heart rate drops during a dive, and its blood circulation changes. Although its brain continues to receive a full supply of blood, the whale's muscles and other, less essential parts of its body are no longer supplied with blood. Only the whale's brain gets oxygen from its blood during a dive.

Blood volume is greater
A whale has a larger amount of blood than a land mammal so it can store a larger amount of oxygen.

Brain

Lungs

Aorta (major artery)

Muscle

Muscles store more oxygen
The whale stores oxygen in its muscles. The oxygen is bound to myoglobin, a substance that picks up oxygen in the lungs, stores it in the muscles, and releases it when it needs to. The whale's muscles contain levels of myoglobin up to 10 times higher than those present in human muscles. This means that a whale's muscles can work during a dive despite their restricted blood supply.

Muscles use energy differently
A whale's muscles can obtain energy from the food the whale eats for a long period of time without the use of oxygen. Evidence also shows that a whale's tissues are less sensitive to carbon dioxide buildup than are those of land mammals, including humans.

Heart

On the surface
A whale's respiratory system is remarkably efficient at ridding its body of carbon dioxide and taking in oxygen when it surfaces after a dive. The whale "pants" through its blowhole. About 90 percent of the air in a whale's lungs is replaced with each breath. Land mammals, including humans, replace only 20 to 33 percent of the air in their lungs with each breath.

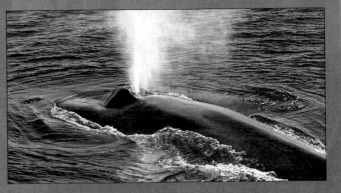

ATMOSPHERIC PRESSURE AND BREATHING

The weight of air pressing down on the Earth is called atmospheric pressure or air pressure. Air pressure, measured in millimeters of mercury (mm Hg), changes at different altitudes. At sea level, the pressure of the air you breathe is about 760 mm Hg. Because this is the average pressure at sea level on the Earth, it is the pressure to which the human body has adapted. A person can survive while breathing air at lower and higher altitudes, but problems can occur if the resultant change in air pressure is too great or if it occurs too quickly.

High altitudes

At high altitudes, the pressure of the air is lower than at sea level. There is less oxygen in the air, reducing the supply of oxygen that passes from your lungs to your blood. If you ascend gradually, your body can adjust to altitudes over 20,000 feet by increasing the number of oxygen-carrying red blood cells it produces. But ascending rapidly to altitudes above 10,000 feet (or sometimes to only 8,000 feet) can cause symptoms of oxygen deficiency, which is also called altitude sickness (see at right). These symptoms gradually diminish as the body adapts, but fluid can build up suddenly in the lungs and sometimes in the brain. The person can die quickly unless he or she is immediately taken to a lower altitude.

Avoiding altitude sickness

To prevent altitude sickness, take several days to ascend to any height above 8,000 feet. If you must ascend faster, return to a lower altitude within a few hours. If you become breathless and have a headache, descend immediately. People with heart or lung diseases must be especially cautious because the oxygen levels in their blood are already low.

Symptoms of altitude sickness
The symptoms of altitude sickness can include breathlessness, rapid pulse, fatigue, headache, nausea, and disturbed thought and vision. Climbers, balloonists, and other people who ascend to heights over 8,000 feet and remain overnight are at increased risk for altitude sickness.

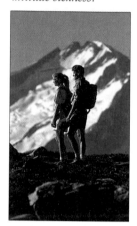

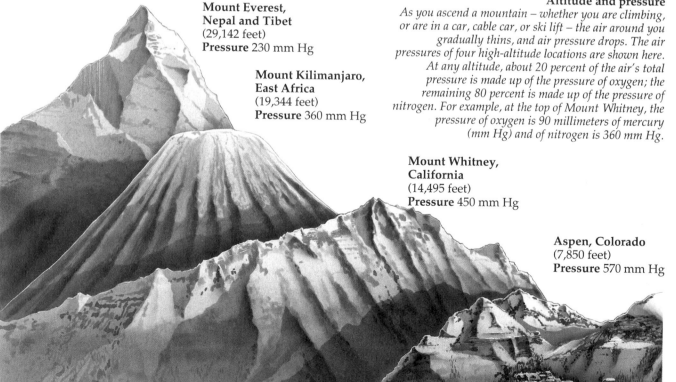

Mount Everest, Nepal and Tibet
(29,142 feet)
Pressure 230 mm Hg

Mount Kilimanjaro, East Africa
(19,344 feet)
Pressure 360 mm Hg

Altitude and pressure
As you ascend a mountain – whether you are climbing, or are in a car, cable car, or ski lift – the air around you gradually thins, and air pressure drops. The air pressures of four high-altitude locations are shown here. At any altitude, about 20 percent of the air's total pressure is made up of the pressure of oxygen; the remaining 80 percent is made up of the pressure of nitrogen. For example, at the top of Mount Whitney, the pressure of oxygen is 90 millimeters of mercury (mm Hg) and of nitrogen is 360 mm Hg.

Mount Whitney, California
(14,495 feet)
Pressure 450 mm Hg

Aspen, Colorado
(7,850 feet)
Pressure 570 mm Hg

Sea level pressure 760 mm Hg

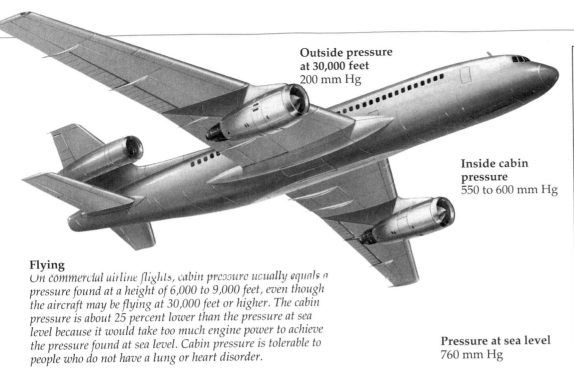

Outside pressure
at 30,000 feet
200 mm Hg

Inside cabin
pressure
550 to 600 mm Hg

Pressure at sea level
760 mm Hg

Flying
On commercial airline flights, cabin pressure usually equals a pressure found at a height of 6,000 to 9,000 feet, even though the aircraft may be flying at 30,000 feet or higher. The cabin pressure is about 25 percent lower than the pressure at sea level because it would take too much engine power to achieve the pressure found at sea level. Cabin pressure is tolerable to people who do not have a lung or heart disorder.

WHO SHOULD NOT FLY?

If you have a lung disorder, such as chronic bronchitis, talk to your doctor before flying. The oxygen levels in your blood are slightly lower than normal. The cabin pressure in an aircraft has a lower oxygen pressure than exists at sea level. This reduced pressure can cause your blood oxygen level to fall low enough to cause severe respiratory problems.

Under water

Scuba divers breathe air at high pressures. Pressure increases rapidly the deeper under water the diver descends. Scuba gear must supply air to a diver's lungs at the same pressure as the external pressure of the water on his or her chest. The deeper a diver goes, the greater the pressure of the air he or she inhales.

When a person inhales air at a pressure four or five times greater than the surface pressure (at about 100 to 130 feet under water), the concentration of nitrogen in the person's blood gradually rises to four or five times the concentration at sea level. This elevated concentration of nitrogen can affect the person's nervous system, causing a slowing of mental functioning called nitrogen narcosis, also known as "rapture of the deep." Judgment becomes impaired, and divers can exhaust their air supply or descend farther instead of surfacing. This phenomenon becomes more pronounced as the diver continues to descend.

Other effects of changes in pressure include decompression sickness ("THE BENDS"; see above right) and pulmonary barotrauma (see right). Both conditions require immediate treatment in a recompression chamber.

"The bends"
The nitrogen in the air that a diver inhales at a great depth gradually saturates the diver's body tissues. If the diver ascends too rapidly, there is not enough time for the nitrogen to leave the tissues. Instead, it can form bubbles, leading to decompression sickness – "the bends." The effects of this condition can range from joint pain to nervous system damage or a stroke.

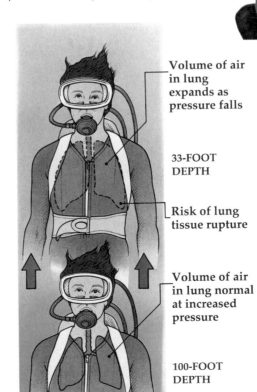

Volume of air
in lung
expands as
pressure falls

**33-FOOT
DEPTH**

Risk of lung
tissue rupture

Volume of air
in lung normal
at increased
pressure

**100-FOOT
DEPTH**

Pulmonary barotrauma
If a scuba diver at a depth of 100 feet takes a deep breath and then ascends without exhaling, the air in the lungs expands rapidly as the external water pressure drops. By the time he or she ascends to a depth of 33 feet, the air occupies twice its original volume. This expansion can cause lung tissue to rupture, a very serious condition called pulmonary barotrauma or a "burst lung." The person experiences immediate breathing difficulty and begins to cough up blood. A diver can easily avoid the condition by consciously exhaling during an ascent.

CHAPTER TWO

RESPIRATORY HEALTH

BECAUSE BREATHING IS largely an unconscious process, we tend to take it for granted. Only when breathing becomes difficult does a person begin to notice the factors that can affect his or her respiratory system. In fact, you can do little to improve an already healthy respiratory system. But you can avoid hazards to your lungs and airways. Cigarette smoking is the single greatest cause of respiratory disease. Smoking causes one in every six deaths and accounts for 87 percent of all lung cancer deaths in the US. An estimated 53,000 deaths each year result from the inhalation of smoke by nonsmokers, called passive smoking. In fact, the "sidestream" smoke generated by smoldering cigarettes between puffs contains higher amounts of toxic and cancer-causing chemicals than the smoke inhaled through a cigarette by a smoker. Smokers pollute not only their own lungs but also the atmosphere around them, placing the health of other people at risk.

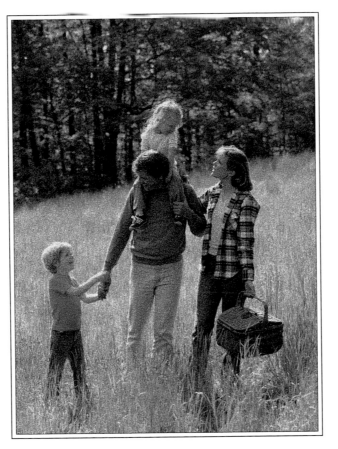

Many lung diseases are caused by inhaling polluted or contaminated air. But unhealthy air is found not only in smog-ridden cities. It can also surround us at home, in the office, and even in rural areas. Indoor pollutants include tobacco smoke, ozone from copying machines and laser printers, vapors from cleaning materials, dust mites that live in carpets, and animal dander (flakes of skin from dogs, cats, and other animals). Because people spend so much of their time indoors, especially children, older people, and the chronically ill, indoor air pollution is a legitimate concern.

To combat the pollution of indoor air, make sure that ventilation is adequate in your home and workplace. Do not allow people to smoke in your home, car, or office. Cut down on the use of products that produce noxious chemical fumes, such as paint thinners and cleaning fluids. Air purifiers have recently become available for the home. Although their benefits are unproven, their popularity reflects our growing concern about indoor air pollution. Certain occupations, such as coal mining and working with asbestos dust, are proven hazards to respiratory health. Medical experts think that many other substances people use at work, such as pesticides and organic dusts, can also pose a hazard when they are inhaled. By minimizing your exposure to air pollutants, you can safeguard your respiratory health. This chapter explores the ways unhealthy air can damage your respiratory system. It also discusses snoring and a respiratory disorder called sleep apnea.

THE AIR YOU BREATHE

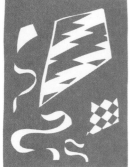

U NLESS BREATHING becomes difficult, you are not usually aware of the process. You probably also take for granted the invisible substance surrounding you – air – that is so vital to life. Most people become aware of the air they breathe only when it smells bad or is irritating, or when it is especially fresh.

When you breathe air, you absorb not only oxygen but also many other gases and particles of matter contained in the air. Some of them can irritate your airways, damage your lungs, and affect your general health.

COMPOSITION OF AIR

At sea level and in dry weather, air consists mainly of two gases. Oxygen makes up about 21 percent of air and nitrogen accounts for about 78 percent. The remainder consists of small amounts of argon and carbon dioxide; trace amounts of gases such as helium, hydrogen, neon, krypton, xenon, and radon; and varying amounts of water vapor.

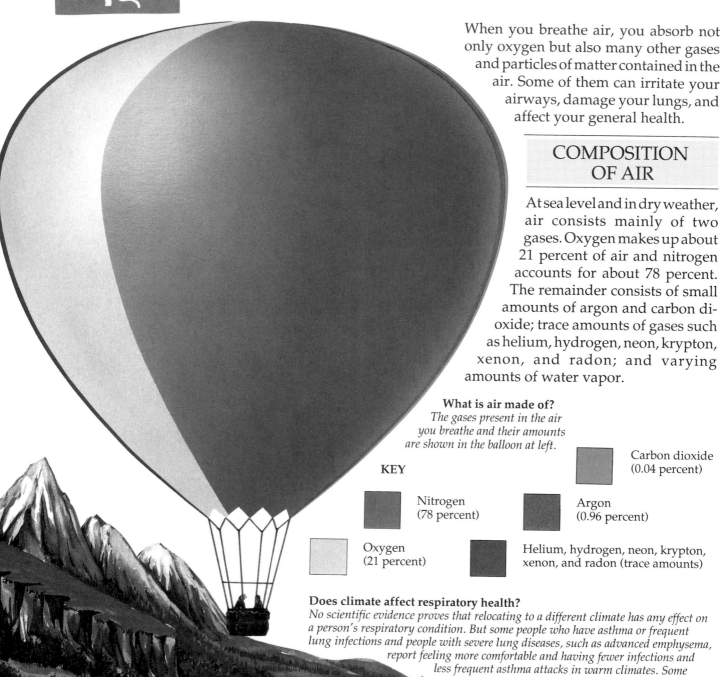

What is air made of?
The gases present in the air you breathe and their amounts are shown in the balloon at left.

KEY

Nitrogen
(78 percent)

Oxygen
(21 percent)

Carbon dioxide
(0.04 percent)

Argon
(0.96 percent)

Helium, hydrogen, neon, krypton, xenon, and radon (trace amounts)

Does climate affect respiratory health?
No scientific evidence proves that relocating to a different climate has any effect on a person's respiratory condition. But some people who have asthma or frequent lung infections and people with severe lung diseases, such as advanced emphysema, report feeling more comfortable and having fewer infections and less frequent asthma attacks in warm climates. Some people prefer warm, dry regions, such as the southwestern US. Others prefer warm, damp regions, such as the southeastern US.

Animal dander
Animal dander – the flakes of skin from dogs and cats – is a common trigger of respiratory allergic reactions. The photograph at right shows animal dander clinging to hairs (magnified 300 times).

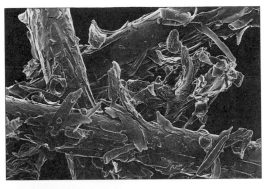

PARTICLES IN THE AIR YOU BREATHE

Countless invisible particles are present in the air you breathe. These particles can include specks of soot and dust; microscopic pieces of dirt, rock, and metal; airborne bacteria and fungal spores; viruses contained in water droplets; house-dust mites; and pollens and other allergens (substances that cause allergic reactions). Air can also contain potentially harmful chemicals, gases, and fumes from industrial, domestic, and naturally occurring sources.

Because the surface area of your alveoli (the tiny air sacs in your lungs) is so extensive (about 260 square feet if they were flattened and spread out), your lungs are more exposed to the environment than is any other part of your body, including your skin. Many particles in the air come into close contact with the alveoli or with the lining of the smaller conducting airways and can cause lung damage. Dissolved particles and chemicals can also get into your bloodstream, ultimately affecting your general health.

Allergens in the air

Allergic reactions include asthma attacks (see ASTHMA on page 92), hay fever caused by airborne pollen (see above left), and allergic rhinitis, a disorder similar to hay fever but occurring throughout the year. Symptoms of allergic rhinitis include a runny nose, sneezing, and postnasal drip (secretions from the sinus cavities and nose that drip down the back of the throat), often accompanied by scratchy, bloodshot eyes. Doctors think allergic rhinitis may be caused by house dust, various types of molds, animal dander, and other allergens in the air. Scientists have recently discovered that the bodies of dead cockroaches contain a chemical that triggers allergies and asthma. When the cockroach bodies decompose, tiny particles become suspended in the air and can be inhaled.

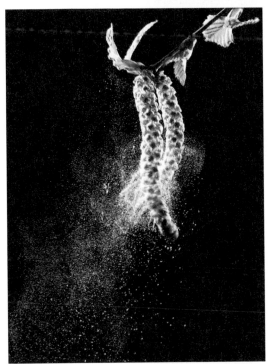

Airborne allergens
Common airborne allergens include ragweed pollen grains, grass and tree pollen grains (shown left), mold spores, various dusts, animal dander, bird feathers, and house-dust mites.

Irritating smoke
Smoke from fires, including those produced by burning leaves, can be irritating to your throat and eyes. The burning of leaves in the autumn is banned in many states because it raises the level of atmospheric pollution.

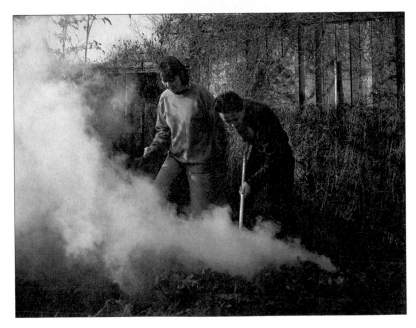

URBAN AIR POLLUTION

City air contains a number of pollutants produced by motor vehicle exhaust and industrial emissions. These pollutants can be extremely irritating and can worsen lung or heart disorders.

Main types of air pollution

Five types of pollutants account for 98 percent of all air pollution. They include substances produced from motor vehicle emissions, such as carbon monoxide, hydrocarbons (solvents and diesel and gasoline vapors), and oxides of nitrogen. Pollution may also be caused by substances produced by burning fossil fuels, such as coal, natural gas, and crude oil. These pollutants include sulfur oxides (including sulfur dioxide) and particles of matter suspended in the air.

Other pollutants include mineral particles, such as powdered coal; vapors, such as formaldehyde; aerosols from spraying pesticides and herbicides; and irritant gases, such as sulfuric acid. Ozone is also a major pollutant in the US during the summer months.

What is ozone?

Ozone is a chemically unstable form of oxygen that can be beneficial or harmful. In the upper parts of the atmosphere (the ozone layer), ozone screens out the sun's most harmful radiation. But when ozone accumulates close to the Earth's surface, it can be a dangerous pollutant that can damage lung tissue. Ozone forms in the lower part of the atmosphere when the byproducts of fossil fuel combustion react in the presence of sunlight. This process commonly occurs in areas of heavy traffic during hot, sunny weather.

EFFECTS OF POLLUTION ON YOUR LUNGS

Many of the pollutants in the air you breathe come into direct contact with your lungs. These pollutants can cause lung damage and increase your susceptibility to lung infections such as pneumonia. Pollutants can also irritate your airways and cause coughing. Allergic or asthmatic reactions can occur in susceptible people. A small proportion, about 2 percent or less, of lung cancers may be caused by air pollution.

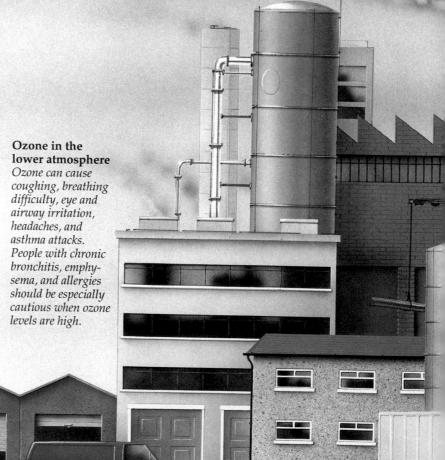

Smoggy cities
Despite strict pollution-control laws, heavy smog still occurs in many large US cities. For example, in Boston, people with lung or heart disease were advised to stay home on more than 20 days in 1989.

Ozone in the lower atmosphere
Ozone can cause coughing, breathing difficulty, eye and airway irritation, headaches, and asthma attacks. People with chronic bronchitis, emphysema, and allergies should be especially cautious when ozone levels are high.

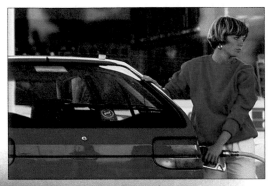

Cleaning up automobile exhaust
Although automobile exhaust still contributes to air pollution, the air has become substantially cleaner since US law mandated the use of unleaded gasoline and required manufacturers to install catalytic converters on cars. Catalytic converters use the metal platinum to convert some substances in automobile exhaust into harmless products, such as water and carbon dioxide.

Major air pollutants
The major pollutants present in urban air are sulfur oxides and small particles of matter suspended in the air from burning fossil fuels, as well as nitrogen oxides, carbon monoxide, and hydrocarbons from motor vehicle emissions.

Smog

The term "smog" originally referred to a combination of smoke, chemical pollutants, and fog. But people commonly use the term to refer to photochemical smog, caused by chemical reactions that occur between strong sunlight and motor vehicle emissions, without the presence of smoke or fog. Other urban air pollutants, such as ozone and nitrogen dioxide, may also contribute to photochemical smog.

ACID RAIN

Excessively acidic precipitation caused by environmental factors is called acid rain. It forms when water droplets in the air combine with chemical pollutants. Rain, snow, or mist can carry these pollutants many miles from their source. Sulfur dioxide forms about 65 percent of the pollutants in acid rain and nitrogen oxides form about 30 percent. Hydrocarbons and ozone in the lower part of the atmosphere also contribute to acid rain. Toxic substances dissolved in acid rain can be inhaled. The sulfur dioxide in acid rain may contribute to respiratory diseases by damaging lung tissue. Acid rain also affects the environment, causing soil infertility, the death of trees, and poisoning of lakes and rivers.

WHAT IS A TEMPERATURE INVERSION?
Weather conditions in some cities can cause an atmospheric temperature inversion. When this happens, the air temperature rises with increasing altitude instead of decreasing as it normally does. Pollutants, which usually rise and become dispersed in the upper atmosphere, remain near the ground and can reach high levels. Temperature inversions can seriously affect people who have respiratory illnesses. Deaths of older people and those with chronic illnesses can increase during such conditions. In 1952 in London, England, about 4,000 people died during periods of temperature inversion.

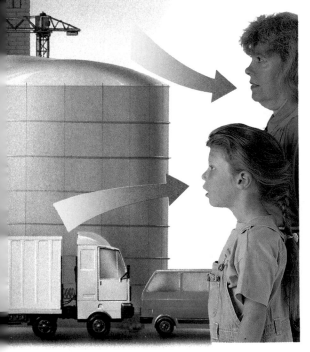

Is the country healthier than the city?
Pollution levels in rural areas have not been thoroughly studied. But pollutants such as insecticides and herbicides that are sprayed on crops are more prevalent in the country than in the city. Some farm workers have experienced respiratory problems after inhaling dust produced during grain transport and storage. No evidence exists to prove that the country is an environment free of respiratory hazards.

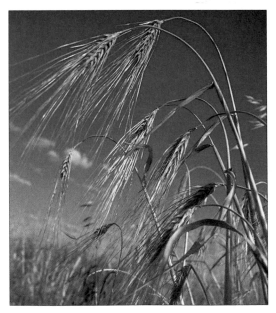

INDOOR AIR QUALITY

Indoor air quality is important because people spend so much of their time indoors. The elderly, the very young, and the chronically ill spend the most time indoors. A number of pollutants can affect the quality of indoor air.

Energy conservation efforts have ensured that today's homes and offices are better insulated against drafts than in the past. But airtight windows and doors reduce the amount of air that circulates through your house. Indoor pollutants range from chemicals such as formaldehyde to fungi and tobacco smoke. In homes or offices that are not adequately ventilated, indoor pollutants can accumulate to unhealthy levels.

AIR POLLUTION IN YOUR HOME

Air pollutants inside your home can originate outside or be generated indoors. Some pollutants can cause or aggravate allergies, such as asthma, hay fever, and allergic rhinitis. Others can lead to lung disorders or infections, or to conditions that affect your general health. The most common sources of indoor pollution can make the air quality in your home poor enough to affect your health.

COMMON AIR POLLUTANTS IN HOMES

● **Tobacco smoke**
People who inhale other people's cigarette smoke are at increased risk of lung cancer, heart attacks, allergies, and chest infections.

● **Automobile exhaust from attached garages**
Poisonous carbon monoxide fumes can enter the house from cracks in floors and walls if you let the car run inside the garage.

● **Radon**
Radon is a radioactive gas that is naturally formed in the ground. It has been detected in the basements of some homes. High levels of radon have caused death from lung cancer in some uranium miners, but no scientific evidence has linked lung cancer with radon exposure among the general public.

● **Burning fuels**
Carbon monoxide from burned fuel such as gas, oil, kerosene, or coal used in stoves can build up in poorly ventilated rooms, causing drowsiness and headaches. High levels of this odorless gas can kill without warning.

● **Hobbies and home improvement**
Many substances used in hobby and home improvement activities can be hazardous. Examples include solvents in glues, fumes from paint, and chemicals in paint strippers. Benzene, found in paint thinner, may cause cancer and may also adversely affect the body's blood-forming system.

● **Microorganisms in air-control devices**
Poorly maintained air-conditioning and heating systems, humidifiers, and dehumidifiers can harbor bacteria and fungi. Clean the filters in your humidifier frequently to avoid the growth of fungi that can cause asthma.

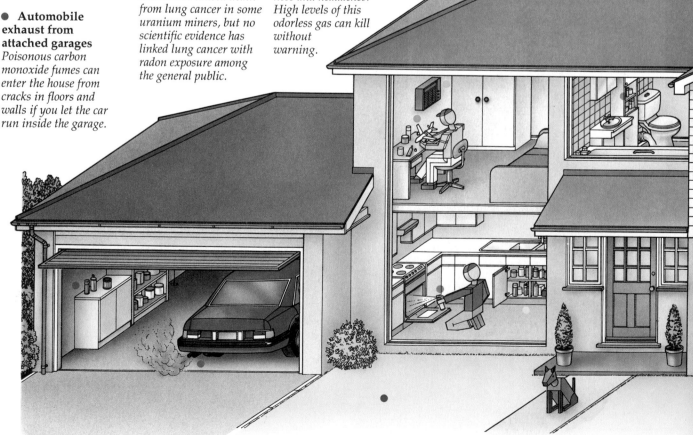

● House dust and airborne allergens

House dust may contain fabric fibers, bacteria, fungal spores, animal dander and hairs, feathers, particles and saps of plants, grass, and tiny insects called house-dust mites. These potential allergens are so common that you cannot easily avoid them, but frequent dusting and vacuuming can reduce their presence.

● Household cleaning materials

Vapors from ammonia and bleach can be irritating when inhaled. Avoid combining cleaning products, which can release harmful vapors.

● Asbestos

With only a few exceptions, every person with a proven asbestos-related disease acquired it at work rather than at home. The most common use of asbestos in older homes is as insulation for pipes or furnaces. Do not try to remove asbestos insulation or other asbestos-containing products from your home. The process of removal releases asbestos fibers into the air, exposing family members to high concentrations of the fibers. Flaking asbestos-containing materials should be sealed by a professional.

● Aerosol cans

Aerosol containers of liquids such as hair spray, air freshener, deodorant, oven cleaner, and insect repellant can release toxic or irritating chemicals.

● Pesticides

Pet flea collars, flea dusts, insect repellants, and rodent-, termite-, and roach-killing products contain highly toxic chemicals. Use these products only when needed and follow package directions.

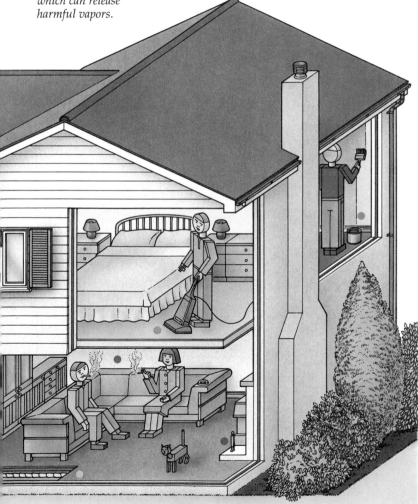

IMPROVE THE AIR QUALITY IN YOUR HOME

◆ Prohibit tobacco smoking in your home or restrict it to one well-ventilated room.

◆ If you suspect asbestos fibers are circulating in your home, have the air tested. Seek advice about removal from your local health department or the regional US Environmental Protection Agency office.

◆ If anyone in your family has allergies, keep the house, especially the bedrooms, as dust-free as possible. Your doctor may recommend that you not keep pets with fur or feathers. Avoid sleeping on feather pillows and choose area rugs or bare floors instead of wall-to-wall carpeting. Eliminate unnecessary items that gather dust.

◆ Open windows regularly to ensure adequate ventilation. Make sure that mechanical ventilation systems are working properly, that fireplaces are swept regularly, and that flues do not become blocked.

◆ Do not inhale the fumes of dangerous substances, such as glues or paint strippers. Use these substances outdoors or near an open window.

◆ Clean heating and air-conditioning filters regularly. Keep humidifier reservoirs and filters clean.

◆ Although the medical benefits of air purifiers have not been proven, you may wish to try them. Mechanical filters and electronic air cleaners remove airborne particles but some produce ozone. Some air cleaners that have activated charcoal remove pollutant gases.

◆ Minimize the use of products dispensed in aerosol cans, such as some hair sprays, oven cleaners, and insect repellents.

AIR POLLUTION IN THE OFFICE

Poor-quality air in an office can adversely affect the health and productivity of employees. The annual cost to business may run in the millions of dollars.

Many newly constructed buildings in the US have heating, ventilation, and air-conditioning systems that control the quality of indoor air. These systems are designed to reduce pollutants, such as dust and particles of matter, to an acceptable level and to provide a comfortable temperature and level of humidity in which to work. Windows in many newer buildings cannot be opened. While ensuring energy efficiency, such building construction allows pollutants to accumulate in recirculated air.

Sources of office pollution

The air in many offices contains gases (such as ozone, carbon monoxide, and nitrogen oxides) produced by photocopiers, laser printers, and solvents contained in products such as typing correction fluid. Microorganisms can also multiply in improperly maintained building ventilation, humidifying, and air-conditioning systems and water-cooling towers. Air circulation systems can distribute these microorganisms, along with particles of dust and other matter, causing health problems.

Photocopiers and laser printers
Good ventilation is especially important near photocopiers and laser printers because these machines produce noxious gases. Ideally, these machines should be located in a separate room in which employees do not spend long periods of time. If this separation is impossible, the machines should be placed in a large, well-ventilated office as far away as possible from desks and other working areas.

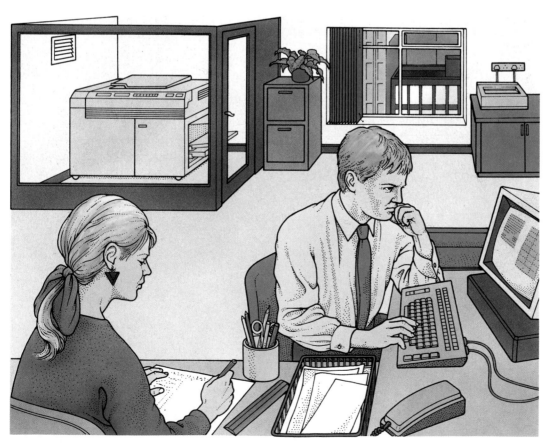

IMPROVING THE QUALITY OF OFFICE AIR
To improve the quality of air in an office, an employer must control the sources of pollutants. Employers must also increase or improve ventilation and possibly use air-cleaning devices. Smoking should not be allowed in an office building or should be restricted to an area outside the building because of the dangers of secondhand smoke. If you or others in your office seem to be sick frequently with no clearly identifiable cause, air quality may be the culprit. Discuss the problem and possible solutions with your employer.

Sick-building syndrome
When symptoms of illness seem related to working or living in a particular building, but no identifiable cause is found, the condition may be attributed to "sick-building syndrome." Symptoms of sick-building syndrome include dry mucous membranes; eye, nose, and throat irritation; headaches; allergies; minor infections; malaise (a general feeling of being sick); and fatigue.

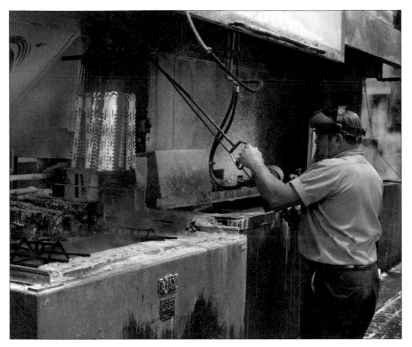

AIR QUALITY PROBLEMS IN THE WORKPLACE

The materials people work with can generate hazardous substances. House painters can inhale toluene in paint, which can cause asthma, or mercury vapor, which can cause headaches, mood swings, nervous system damage, or death. Farm workers can inhale allergens present in dusts from animals or grains; infectious organisms from the dried dusts of animal feces or droppings; or chemicals found in insecticides, herbicides, and fungicides. Construction workers can breathe in dust and harmful substances, such as asbestos fibers, found in many types of building, insulation, and fireproofing materials; metal fumes created during welding; fumes from paint, wood preservatives, sealants, and waterproofing materials; and pesticides used for timber treatment. During drilling, dental workers can inhale silica particles, which can cause the scarring lung disease called silicosis (see page 112). People who work at dry cleaners can inhale the solvent tetrachloroethylene, which can cause dizziness, drowsiness, and liver damage.

Exposure to dangerous fumes
Adequate ventilation is important when people are working with toxic or irritant fumes from hot metals.

SAFETY PRECAUTIONS

Be aware of possible health hazards in your workplace. Follow the health and safety regulations that apply where you work and use protective equipment or clothing. Some industries require that you wear protective clothing and headgear. Avoid working with potentially harmful substances, such as asbestos, or in a poorly ventilated place. If you think your working environment does not meet the legal safety requirements, talk to your employer.

ASK YOUR DOCTOR
AIR QUALITY

Q I ride my bike to work along a busy highway. I am worried that the traffic exhaust fumes could affect my health. Should I wear a mask or change my route to work?

A Try taking another route to work. Wearing a paper mask like the ones used by floor sanders will not protect you from vehicle exhaust. The canister-type masks that provide better protection would probably be unwieldy during a prolonged period of vigorous biking.

Q Why does my asthma improve when I go skiing? Is the air quality better in the mountains?

A At high altitudes, the air is cold and dry and the environment is hostile to the house-dust mite to which you might be allergic. You may also be staying in a house or hotel that is free of pet dander and air pollutants. In some people with asthma, attacks are triggered by cold weather, so going to a ski resort is not the remedy for everyone.

Q What exactly is carbon monoxide and why is it so dangerous for people to inhale?

A Carbon monoxide is a gas produced by incomplete fuel combustion that is present in automobile exhaust and cigarette smoke. If inhaled at high levels, it can severely reduce the blood's ability to carry oxygen to your body's cells. A person will eventually lose consciousness and die if exposed to carbon monoxide for a long period. The gas is odorless and colorless and can be emitted by faulty home heating systems. Have your heating system inspected each winter.

HAZARDS OF SMOKING

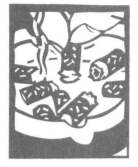

EACH TIME YOU INHALE a puff of cigarette smoke, you draw poisonous chemicals into your airways and lungs. Your bloodstream absorbs many of these chemicals and transports them to all parts of your body. There are more than 4,000 different compounds in tobacco smoke, many of them poisonous or able to cause genetic mutations. Researchers have identified 43 chemicals in tobacco smoke that can cause cancer.

Smoking is the top preventable cause of death in the US. Researchers have cited smoking as the major cause of lung cancer and of chronic bronchitis and emphysema (together called chronic obstructive pulmonary disease). Smoking also causes oral and esophageal cancer and contributes to heart disease and stroke.

Smoking is the nation's most widespread form of drug dependency. Most people who smoke begin when they are too young to make decisions that will affect their future health. But antismoking efforts have succeeded in reducing the prevalence of smoking from 40 percent of all adults in the US in 1965 to 28 percent in 1988.

Damage to the lungs
A person who smokes 20 cigarettes every day inhales smoke about 70,000 times a year. With every puff, the person's airways and lungs are exposed to noxious chemicals.

INCREASED CANCER RISK

Smoking not only causes deaths from lung cancer but also increases the risk of cancer of the mouth, lips, tongue, throat, esophagus, stomach, and bladder. Cancer is not the only risk. Smoking also contributes to the development of high blood pressure and heart disease.

Increased susceptibility
People who smoke increase the susceptibility of their lungs to damage from other pollutants that irritate the respiratory system, such as smog.

TOBACCO SMOKE

Tobacco smoke kills cells that clear debris from the lungs and paralyzes the hairlike projections that line and protect the airways. Smoking also alters lung enzyme activity, destroying air sacs in the lungs, which leads to emphysema.

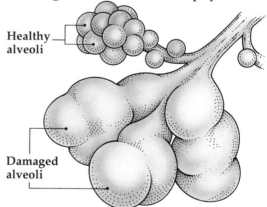

Healthy alveoli

Damaged alveoli

Emphysema from smoking
Emphysema damages the alveoli (small air sacs) in the lungs. They ultimately merge to form fewer, larger air sacs. This process causes a reduction in the lung's surface area and less efficient transfer of oxygen to the bloodstream. Emphysema is almost always caused by tobacco smoking.

Nicotine

Nicotine is the substance in tobacco smoke that makes smoking addictive. Although nicotine is less destructive than other poisons in cigarette smoke, doctors call this substance a cocarcinogen – meaning that nicotine works in combination with other substances in cigarette smoke to cause cancer.

Tar

Tar is the sticky brown residue that forms when tobacco is burned. It consists of many different chemicals, primarily hydrocarbons. Hydrocarbons can cause mutations of genes and are powerful carcinogens (cancer-causing substances). Researchers have established that tar is a direct cause of lung cancer.

Other poisonous chemicals

Other chemicals in tobacco smoke include arsenic, ammonia, formaldehyde, lead, benzene (also found in paint thinner), and vinyl chloride (also used in the production of plastics). These poisons stimulate excessive production of mucus, which clogs the airways. This obstruction makes the smoker cough and causes bronchitis and other disorders.

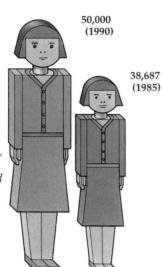

Lung cancer in women
The increase in deaths from lung cancer among women who smoke has made lung cancer the leading cause of cancer deaths in women. From 1985 to 1990, lung cancer deaths in women increased by 30 percent.

50,000 (1990)

38,687 (1985)

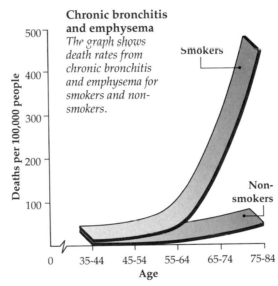

Chronic bronchitis and emphysema
The graph shows death rates from chronic bronchitis and emphysema for smokers and non-smokers.

Deaths per 100,000 people

Smokers

Non-smokers

Age — 35-44, 45-54, 55-64, 65-74, 75-84

FACTS ABOUT SMOKERS

◆ Smokers are highly susceptible to infection.

◆ Women smokers go through menopause earlier than nonsmoking women.

◆ Smokers have faster heart rates.

◆ Women who smoke during pregnancy have low birthweight babies.

◆ Mothers who smoke are twice as likely to have a child die of sudden infant death syndrome than nonsmoking mothers.

◆ Smokers develop high blood pressure much earlier than nonsmokers with high blood pressure.

PASSIVE SMOKING

Research has shown that passive smoking – inhaling other people's smoke – is a serious health hazard. Smoke emitted from the burning end of a cigarette actually contains higher concentrations of many toxins, such as nicotine and cancer-causing nitrosamines (also used in the production of dyes), than the smoke inhaled through a cigarette by a smoker. Studies have found that:

◆ Children of smokers are twice as likely to be hospitalized for bronchitis and pneumonia in the first year of life than children of nonsmokers.

◆ Almost one fifth of all lung cancers that occur in nonsmokers are caused by passive smoking.

◆ Exposure to cigarette smoke in the home for 25 years can double the risk of lung cancer for a nonsmoker.

◆ Passive smoking worsens asthma, allergies, and heart disease.

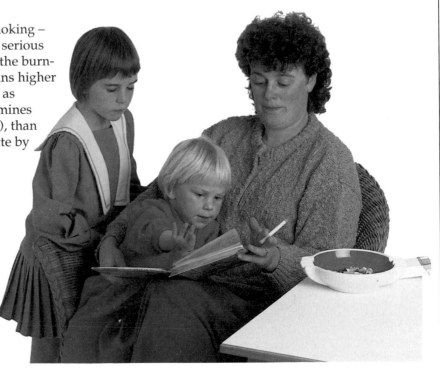

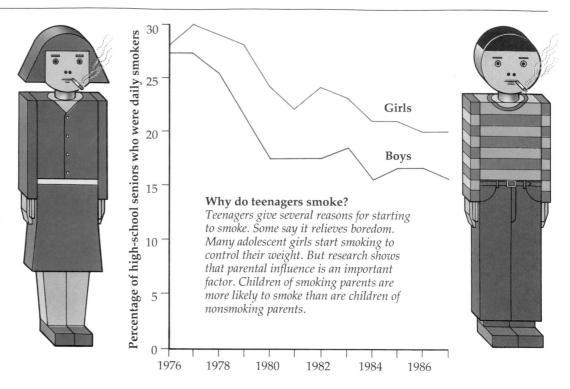

Teenage smokers
The graph at right shows, for the years from 1976 to 1987, the percentages of high-school seniors who were daily smokers. The total number of adolescent smokers fell during this period, but the number of adolescent female smokers remained consistently higher than the number of adolescent male smokers. More recent data show that teenage girls are starting to smoke at increasingly earlier ages. Once they start, females are more likely than males to continue smoking.

Why do teenagers smoke?
Teenagers give several reasons for starting to smoke. Some say it relieves boredom. Many adolescent girls start smoking to control their weight. But research shows that parental influence is an important factor. Children of smoking parents are more likely to smoke than are children of nonsmoking parents.

WHO IS SMOKING?

Although more than 50 million Americans smoke cigarettes, the number of smokers over 20 declined from a high of 40 percent of the adult population in 1965 to 28 percent in 1988. Among men, the percentage who smoke cigarettes peaked at 53 percent in 1964; this figure then declined to 31 percent by 1988. This decline reflects both an increase in the number of men who have quit smoking and a decrease in the number of young men who have started smoking.

The prevalence of smoking is highest among men born in the 1920s and among women born in the 1930s and 1940s.

Women who smoke

Overall, more men than women smoke. But, among people born between 1960 and 1963, more women than men smoke. Since 1977, cigarette smoking has been more common among adolescent girls than among boys. The percentage of women who smoke rose to a peak of 34 percent in 1965. Since then, the decline in smoking among women has been less

dramatic than in men. From 1965 to 1977, the percentage of women smokers remained between 31 and 32 percent and only fell to 26 percent by 1988. The number of women who are quitting smoking is increasing but, unlike men, young women are still starting to smoke at a steady rate.

Smoking increases a woman's risk of lung and heart disease and has a number of other harmful effects. For example, women who smoke have an increased risk of cancer of the cervix. Smoking interacts with birth control pills to boost the risk of heart attacks in women tenfold. Tobacco smoking can also reduce a woman's fertility.

When do people start smoking?
On the average, young men start smoking at about age 17 and young women start at about age 19. The younger a person starts to smoke, the more likely he or she is to continue smoking throughout life.

SMOKELESS TOBACCO

Smokeless tobacco can be purchased as snuff, chewing tobacco, or loose-leaf tobacco in pouches. In the last 20 years, smokeless tobacco use has risen, especially among adolescent boys. In the US, about 4 million young people between the ages of 10 and 20 use smokeless tobacco. About 19 percent of high-school boys report using smokeless tobacco. But less than 2 percent of high-school girls use it in any form.

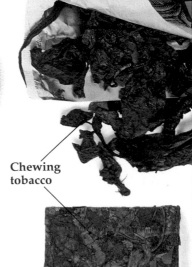
Snuff

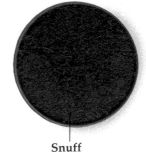
Chewing tobacco

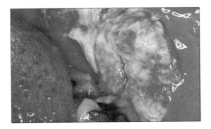

Health hazards of smokeless tobacco
The concentrations of cancer-causing substances in smokeless tobacco are 100 times higher than those found in cigarette, cigar, or pipe tobacco. People who chew tobacco or use snuff are at risk for cancer of the lip, cheek (shown at left), or tongue; gum disease; and tooth decay. Smokeless tobacco use can cause nicotine addiction and increases the likelihood of cigarette smoking.

RISKS OF SMOKING DURING PREGNANCY

When a pregnant woman smokes, the hazardous substances in tobacco smoke pass into her blood and travel to the placenta. Some of these substances reduce the transfer of oxygen and nutrients across the placenta into the fetus's circulation.

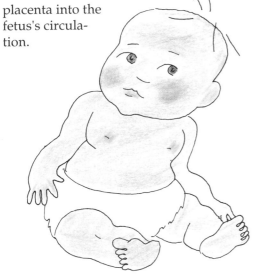

Dangers before and after birth
Smoking during pregnancy increases the risks of miscarriage, stillbirth, and newborn death and lowers the average birth weight. Research suggests that smoking during pregnancy can adversely affect the child's intellectual performance as well. Sudden infant death syndrome is more common in babies born to women who smoke during pregnancy.

WHO HAS QUIT?

Nearly half of all living adults who ever smoked have quit. The trend toward not smoking has steadily gained followers since 1966. Younger people are more likely to try to quit smoking than are older people, and women are more likely to make the attempt than are men. But men who quit are more likely to abstain for 5 years or more. The longer a person can go without a cigarette, the less likely he or she is to begin smoking again.

Benefits of quitting

People who quit smoking add years to their life. Many of the risks are greatly reduced 1 to 5 years after quitting. For example, 1 year after quitting, the risk of heart disease from smoking drops by half. Fifteen years after quitting, the smoking-related health risks of ex-smokers match the risks of people who have never smoked. By quitting smoking, a person reduces the risk of lung cancer and other cancers, long-term lung diseases (such as chronic bronchitis and emphysema) and other respiratory illnesses, coronary heart disease, and stroke.

CIGAR AND PIPE SMOKING

Because cigar and pipe smokers usually inhale less smoke than cigarette smokers, their overall death rates are much lower. But all smokers are at equal risk of death from cancers of the mouth, larynx, and esophagus. The number of men who smoke cigars and pipes has declined substantially since 1964. Today, only about 6 percent of men smoke cigars and about 4 percent smoke pipes.

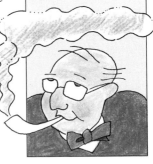

QUITTING SMOKING

More than 70 percent of smokers say that they would like to quit smoking. Ninety-five percent of former smokers have quit without formal help and most look back on the process as having been easier than they expected. But a smoker will not succeed unless he or she has made a firm decision to quit. Many types of programs have been designed to help.

Getting ready

The first step toward quitting smoking is to motivate yourself. Think of the reasons you should not smoke. It's bad for your health and your appearance. It annoys other people. It makes your breath, hair, and clothes smell bad. It costs a lot of money. Analyze your habit carefully so that you know exactly when you smoke and what prompts you to light up.

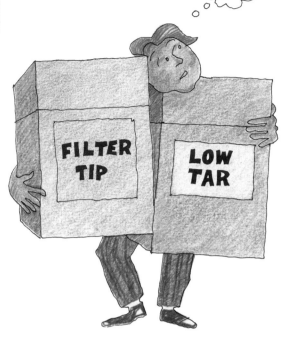

Low-tar and filter-tip cigarettes
Some people think that low-tar, low-nicotine, or filter-tip cigarettes are less hazardous than ordinary ones. But switching to these types of cigarettes will not reduce your risk of respiratory disease because the amount of dangerous chemicals in the smoke these cigarettes generate is reduced only slightly.

COLD TURKEY
Some people find that the best way to quit smoking is to stop cold, rather than to gradually cut down on smoking. If you decide on this way to quit smoking, it might help to do so when you are on vacation or while you are under lower amounts of stress than usual. Sometimes unfamiliar surroundings can help you break the habit of smoking at certain times of the day or in specific situations, such as during your coffee break at work.

Make a checklist
Write down the reasons you smoke and when you are most likely to light up. Use this list to help avoid the situations in which you tend to smoke.

Taking the plunge

If you can, choose a low-stress time to quit smoking. Carefully plan ahead for the day you quit for good. Begin consciously cutting down on the number of times a day that you smoke.

Change your daily routine so that you can avoid situations in which you tend to smoke. Develop new interests, such

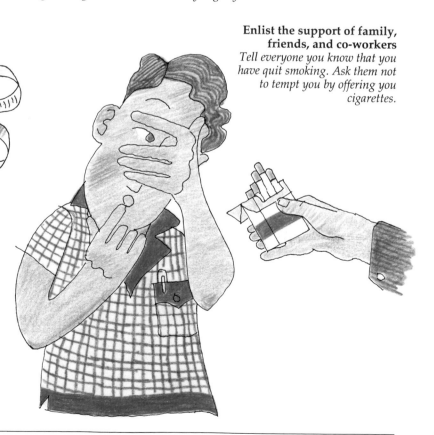

Enlist the support of family, friends, and co-workers
Tell everyone you know that you have quit smoking. Ask them not to tempt you by offering you cigarettes.

as playing cards or putting puzzles together, to keep your hands busy. Tackle those home improvement projects you may have put off. Most importantly, engage in exercise, such as brisk walking, biking, swimming, or jogging. These activities will boost your level of fitness, reduce stress, and help you avoid putting on weight. Eat regular, balanced meals. Be careful if you drink alcohol – it can weaken your willpower.

Substitute something else for the cigarettes
Keep a supply of fresh carrots and celery sticks on hand to munch when you get the urge to smoke. Or chew sugar-free gum. Nicotine gum or nicotine patches, which your doctor can prescribe for you, can help during the first few weeks.

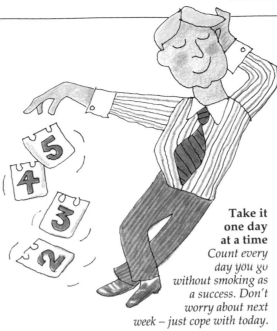

Take it one day at a time
Count every day you go without smoking as a success. Don't worry about next week – just cope with today.

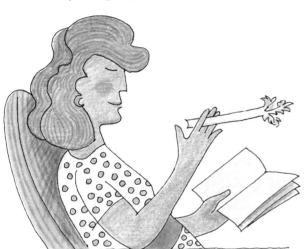

SUPPORT SYSTEMS
You might find it helpful to join a support group for ex-smokers or people who are trying to quit. When you decide to quit smoking, nothing is as important to your success as determination and willpower. When you are in danger of relapsing, support from other people can make the difference between success and failure.

Following through
Most people who try quitting go through the process several times before they quit smoking for good. The most likely time for a relapse occurs about 3 months after you quit, because at this stage you feel confident that you can take or leave smoking at will. If you begin smoking again, remember that a lapse is not complete failure. Get yourself motivated to quit again. The longer you refrain from smoking after the 3-month mark, the less likely you are to begin again.

THE FIRST FEW DAYS AS A NONSMOKER

During the first few days after you quit, the following problems can occur, but they are usually only temporary:

◆ **Cravings to smoke.** Get up and do something. Go for a walk, telephone a friend, or do a crossword puzzle to take your mind off smoking.

◆ **Irritability and mood swings.** Warn your friends and family ahead of time that you might become irritable so they will understand and be helpful.

◆ **Lack of concentration, restlessness, or altered sleep patterns.** Nicotine gum or nicotine patches can help ease these common symptoms of nicotine withdrawal.

◆ **A cough.** Nervous tension may make you cough more in the first few days. Unless you have severe bronchitis, your cough will soon disappear.

◆ **Increased appetite**. Eating should not become a substitute for smoking. If you must nibble, eat fresh fruit and vegetables. Drink at least eight glasses of water a day and get plenty of exercise to work off those few extra pounds.

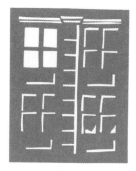

SNORING AND SLEEP APNEA

SNORING CAN RANGE from a low hum to a roar so loud it can awaken someone in the next room. Most snoring is harmless. But occasionally it can signal a condition known as sleep apnea, in which breathing can stop for 10 seconds or more several times each night, waking up the person for brief periods.

Snoring is a recurrent, low-pitched vibration of the soft palate (the flexible tissue at the back of the roof of the mouth) that occurs when people breathe through their mouths and sleep on their backs. Snoring can intensify when you have a cold, a small growth in the nose, enlarged tonsils or adenoids (lymph nodes at the back of the nose), or inflamed nasal passages. Loud snoring that is prolonged and interrupted with gasps and pauses in breathing may indicate a problem such as sleep apnea. Talk to your doctor if your snoring keeps your partner awake, awakens you, or causes symptoms of sleep apnea (see below).

SLEEP APNEA

A person with sleep apnea stops breathing during sleep for more than 10 seconds several times an hour. When breathing stops, oxygen levels in the blood fall, and the brain eventually awakens the sleeper so breathing can resume. These awakenings can prevent the person from getting a good night's sleep. Daytime symptoms include drowsiness, irritability, anxiety, and depression.

Obstructive sleep apnea

Obstructive sleep apnea, also called upper-airway apnea, is a severe but common sleep disorder. In this form of sleep apnea, breathing stops because of blocked airways. The sleeper usually is unaware that the breathing problem has

INFANT APNEA

In infant apnea, pauses of up to 15 seconds occur in a baby's breathing during sleep. Apnea occurs more often in boys than in girls and can often be traced to an infection, an airway obstruction, or a seizure. Often, no cause is apparent. Infant apnea may not be a cause for concern. But if breathing stops for 20 seconds or more, the baby could turn blue and go limp. Although a pinch on the baby's bottom may restore breathing, consult your pediatrician about the problem.

Blocked airways in obstructive sleep apnea
In obstructive sleep apnea, the muscles at the back of the throat collapse, and the surrounding tissue helps block the airway and stop breathing. Enlarged tonsils and adenoids contribute to the problem.

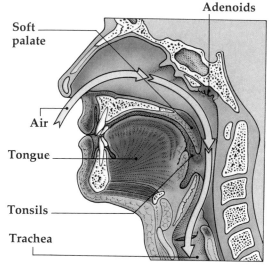

Adenoids

Soft palate

Air

Tongue

Tonsils

Trachea

AWAKE – AIRWAY OPEN

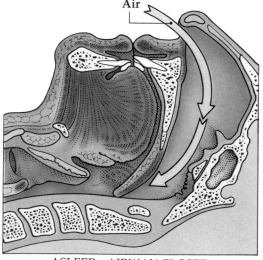

Air

ASLEEP – AIRWAY CLOSED

Falling blood oxygen levels in sleep apnea

Each time the sleeper stops breathing, the amount of oxygen in his or her blood falls (see below), and the person's heart must work harder to compensate. Blood pressure rises and the heart rhythm may become irregular. As the oxygen level continues to fall, the person's diaphragm and chest muscles become stimulated to contract so air can enter the lungs. The person awakens briefly, takes a huge breath, and falls asleep again, only to repeat the pattern later.

Blood oxygen saturation levels

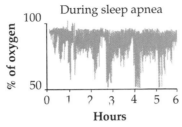

During normal sleep

During sleep apnea

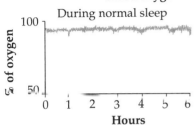

Central sleep apnea

In central sleep apnea, the airways stay open. But for reasons that are unclear, the brain fails to send appropriate nerve signals to the diaphragm and chest muscles, which stop working. Breathing temporarily stops until falling oxygen levels in the blood prompt the sleeper to awaken and begin breathing again. People with central sleep apnea usually complain of sleeping poorly.

occurred. A person with obstructive sleep apnea can stop breathing and partially awaken many times each night. The disorder is common in overweight, middle-aged men, especially if they drink heavily. It can also develop in middle-aged women and in a person who has large tonsils or a small opening to his or her airway. People who take sleeping pills or antihistamines or who drink alcohol before going to bed are also at risk for this condition because the muscles in the upper airway become more relaxed.

Sleep laboratories

If you regularly experience disturbed sleep, you can be tested in a sleep laboratory. Tests are conducted overnight to measure oxygen levels in your blood and the airflow from your nose and mouth. Recordings of your brain waves, your heart rhythm, and the activity of your eye muscles during sleep are also made.

TREATING APNEA AND APNEA-RELATED SNORING

◆ An overweight person's snoring or apnea can be alleviated by losing excess weight.

◆ Cutting down on alcohol consumption and on the use of sleeping pills helps reduce apnea and snoring.

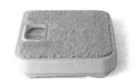

◆ To minimize snoring, people should avoid sleeping on their backs.

◆ The drug protriptyline can help reduce snoring by stimulating the throat muscles to prevent the airway from collapsing.

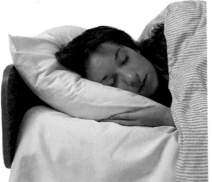

◆ Surgery can be done to remove enlarged tonsils, adenoids, or the rear border of the soft palate, but these procedures do not always successfully treat the apnea or snoring, especially in adults.

◆ A continuous positive airway pressure mask, worn during the night, uses pressure from an air compressor to keep the airway open so that the person does not stop breathing. Doctors use this mask mainly to treat people who have obstructive sleep apnea.

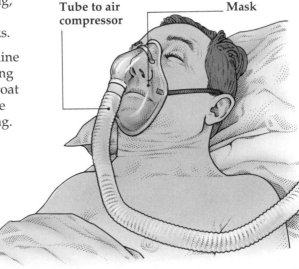

Tube to air compressor

Mask

CHAPTER THREE

SYMPTOMS AND DIAGNOSIS

INTRODUCTION

SYMPTOMS OF RESPIRATORY DISEASE

YOUR DOCTOR'S EXAMINATION

IMAGING THE LUNGS

TESTS AND PROCEDURES

FROM TIME TO TIME, we all experience respiratory system problems. The symptoms of these problems are effectively treated with simple over-the-counter remedies, plenty of fluids, and bed rest. But when symptoms persist or become severe, they can signal a more serious respiratory system disorder. You should consult your doctor whenever you experience symptoms such as unexplained breathlessness, severe chest pain, or coughing up of blood.

Never delay in getting medical help for children, because they can develop serious illnesses very quickly. What may seem like the symptoms of a simple cold can herald an ear infection, measles, or meningitis (inflammation of the membranes that surround the brain and spinal cord). Infections are the most common illnesses in children and young adults. You should always ask your doctor to investigate infections that produce a prolonged or high fever, along with other symptoms (such as breathlessness). A persistent cough in a child can be an early sign of asthma, pertussis (whooping cough), or sinus problems. Adults, especially those over 40, are susceptible to a broad range of respiratory diseases. Older adults have a much higher incidence of lung cancer and blood clots in the lungs.

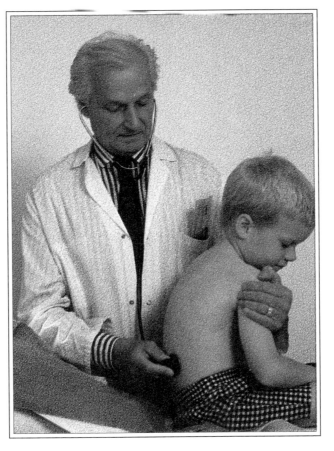

If you see your doctor because of respiratory symptoms, he or she will ask about the onset and persistence of your symptoms. Your doctor will also perform a thorough physical examination and will obtain a chest X-ray. If your doctor suspects an infection, phlegm or blood samples may be taken to identify the organism that caused the infection. If these tests do not produce conclusive results, a technique called bronchoscopy may be performed to obtain phlegm or tissue samples. If the doctor thinks the diagnosis could be asthma, the functioning of your lungs will be tested. Doctors also perform tests that can detect cancerous cells. When the doctor reaches a diagnosis, he or she will prescribe appropriate treatment. If a disease seems serious, the doctor will begin treatment, based on the most likely diagnosis, before test results come back.

This chapter describes some of the most common symptoms of respiratory disease, including difficulty breathing, wheezing, chest pain, and coughing. Later, we discuss the procedures, including the physical examination and diagnostic tests, your doctor follows to diagnose respiratory problems. The chapter explains various imaging techniques, such as chest X-ray and CT scanning, that doctors use to detect lung disorders.

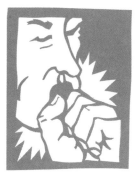

SYMPTOMS OF RESPIRATORY DISEASE

Y OUR BODY CAN function normally for only a few minutes without oxygen, so any disorder that makes you gasp for air can be frightening. Wheezing, coughing, or chest pain can signal a serious respiratory problem. But these symptoms can also be caused by a nonrespiratory disorder, such as heart disease, so you should see your doctor as soon as such symptoms occur.

HOW BREATH-LESS ARE YOU?

When you see your doctor, he or she may ask you questions about the severity of your difficulty breathing, such as:

◆ How far can you walk before you have to stop to catch your breath?

◆ How many stairs can you climb before you have to stop for a breath?

◆ Does the breathlessness affect your job or sex life?

◆ Do you ever feel so breathless that you are afraid you are going to die?

◆ Do you get short of breath when you lie down? If so, how many pillows do you use at night?

Not all respiratory symptoms indicate a severe disorder. For example, a cough can accompany a cold or minor throat irritation from dust or smoke. But other symptoms, such as difficulty breathing, are more likely to result from a serious problem. Your doctor should investigate any unusual or persistent symptoms.

DIFFICULTY BREATHING

Everyone feels breathless after vigorous exercise, but it is not normal to become breathless at rest or after minimal exer-cise. Difficulty breathing can be caused not only by a respiratory condition, but also by underlying heart disease, ane-mia, or a disorder of the brain or nervous system affecting the nerves that control the breathing muscles. During preg-nancy, difficulty breathing can occur when the growing fetus presses against the mother's rib cage. It is also a common symptom of anxiety. Because so many factors can cause breathing problems, you should consult your doctor if you experience shortness of breath from anything other than exertion.

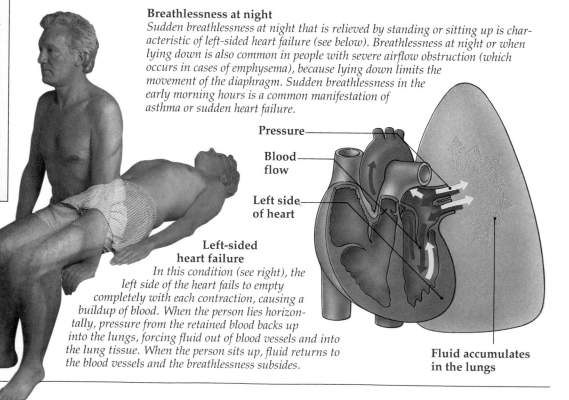

Breathlessness at night
Sudden breathlessness at night that is relieved by standing or sitting up is char-acteristic of left-sided heart failure (see below). Breathlessness at night or when lying down is also common in people with severe airflow obstruction (which occurs in cases of emphysema), because lying down limits the movement of the diaphragm. Sudden breathlessness in the early morning hours is a common manifestation of asthma or sudden heart failure.

Pressure

Blood flow

Left side of heart

Left-sided heart failure
In this condition (see right), the left side of the heart fails to empty completely with each contraction, causing a buildup of blood. When the person lies horizon-tally, pressure from the retained blood backs up into the lungs, forcing fluid out of blood vessels and into the lung tissue. When the person sits up, fluid returns to the blood vessels and the breathlessness subsides.

Fluid accumulates in the lungs

CAUSES OF DIFFICULTY BREATHING

Any condition that affects the flow of air into or out of the lungs, the exchange of oxygen and carbon dioxide inside the lungs, or the circulation of blood through the lungs can be a source of difficulty breathing. The speed with which symptoms develop provides your doctor with clues about the cause.

KEY

■ Symptoms develop slowly over many years
□ Symptoms develop over days or weeks
■ Symptoms develop over a few hours
□ Sudden onset of symptoms

Chronic bronchitis
Persistent inflammation of the airways (usually caused by smoking) leads to a buildup of mucus and a narrowing of the air passages, which impede air flow.

Emphysema
When the alveoli (small air sacs) in the lungs are damaged (usually by smoking), they break down and grow together, reducing the surface area needed for the exchange of oxygen and carbon dioxide.

Scarred lung tissue

Blood clot

Pulmonary embolism
Blood clots become lodged in the blood vessels of the lungs, depriving affected lung tissue of blood, so that the exchange of oxygen and carbon dioxide cannot occur.

Interstitial lung disease
The lungs become distorted, stiffened, and scarred with fibrous tissue. Scarring impairs oxygen transfer and the person feels short of breath.

Lung cancer
A tumor can block a large airway or damage large portions of the lung.

Pneumonia
Infection of the lungs causes inflammation of lung tissue. The air spaces become filled with fluid and pus.

Narrowed air passages

Allergic reaction
An allergic reaction to some substances (called allergens) causes inflammation and narrowing of the air passages (asthma). Examples of common allergens include house-dust mites, pollens, and animal dander.

Pulmonary edema
The pressure of fluid rises in the blood vessels supplying the lungs. Fluid leaks out of the capillaries and fills the air spaces, impairing the exchange of oxygen and carbon dioxide. The condition usually results from heart failure (reduced pumping efficiency).

Pneumothorax (collapsed lung)
A penetrating chest injury or rupture of lung tissue can allow air to enter the space between the membranes that surround the lungs. This air creates increased pressure on the outside of the lung, forcing it to collapse.

Collapsed lung

Air outside lung

61

MONITOR YOUR SYMPTOMS
DIFFICULTY BREATHING

Breathing difficulty, or shortness of breath, is the sensation of not being able to get enough air. A disruption in breathing can threaten the body's vital supply of oxygen. If you notice any of the symptoms mentioned in this chart, seek medical advice promptly. If you also experience wheezing along with shortness of breath, see the WHEEZING chart on page 64.

> **WARNING**
>
> If a person is having severe difficulty breathing, especially if there is a bluish tinge to his or her lips, the situation is an emergency requiring immediate medical attention. Dial 911 or call emergency medical services in your community. While waiting for medical help to arrive, loosen any tight clothing the person is wearing and help him or her sit up.

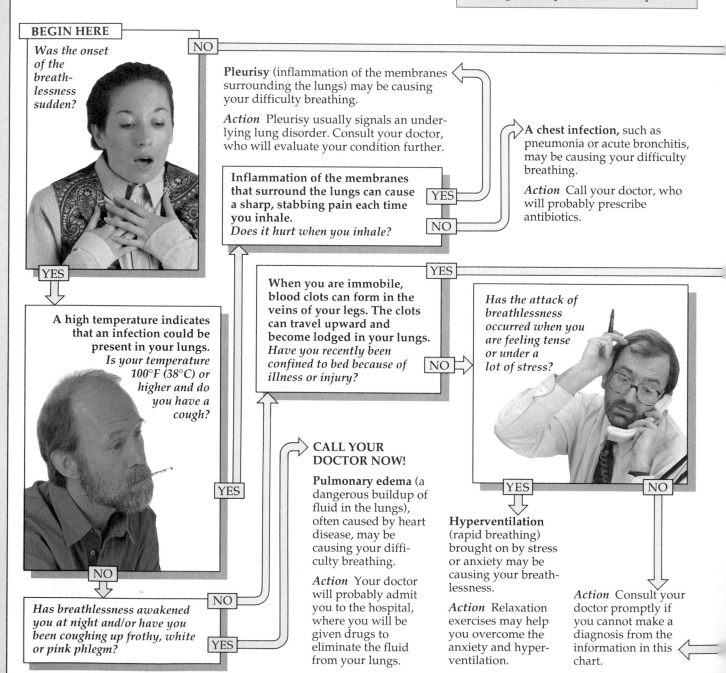

BEGIN HERE

Was the onset of the breathlessness sudden? — NO →

Pleurisy (inflammation of the membranes surrounding the lungs) may be causing your difficulty breathing.

Action Pleurisy usually signals an underlying lung disorder. Consult your doctor, who will evaluate your condition further.

Inflammation of the membranes that surround the lungs can cause a sharp, stabbing pain each time you inhale.
Does it hurt when you inhale? — YES / NO

A chest infection, such as pneumonia or acute bronchitis, may be causing your difficulty breathing.

Action Call your doctor, who will probably prescribe antibiotics.

YES ↓

A high temperature indicates that an infection could be present in your lungs.
Is your temperature 100°F (38°C) or higher and do you have a cough?

When you are immobile, blood clots can form in the veins of your legs. The clots can travel upward and become lodged in your lungs.
Have you recently been confined to bed because of illness or injury? — NO →

Has the attack of breathlessness occurred when you are feeling tense or under a lot of stress? — YES / NO

CALL YOUR DOCTOR NOW!

Pulmonary edema (a dangerous buildup of fluid in the lungs), often caused by heart disease, may be causing your difficulty breathing.

Action Your doctor will probably admit you to the hospital, where you will be given drugs to eliminate the fluid from your lungs.

Hyperventilation (rapid breathing) brought on by stress or anxiety may be causing your breathlessness.

Action Relaxation exercises may help you overcome the anxiety and hyperventilation.

Action Consult your doctor promptly if you cannot make a diagnosis from the information in this chart.

YES ↓

Has breathlessness awakened you at night and/or have you been coughing up frothy, white or pink phlegm? — NO / YES

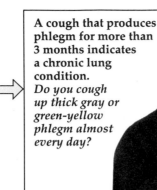

A cough that produces phlegm for more than 3 months indicates a chronic lung condition.
Do you cough up thick gray or green-yellow phlegm almost every day?

NO

Smokers have an increased risk of lung cancer.
Do you smoke and have you lost weight recently and/or coughed up blood-stained phlegm?

YES   NO

YES

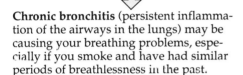

Dusts from such minerals as coal, asbestos, sand, and quartz can produce chronic lung tissue disorders.
Did you ever work in a dusty atmosphere, such as a mine or quarry?

NO   YES

CONSULT YOUR DOCTOR NOW!

Lung cancer is a possible cause of your breathlessness, especially if you are a heavy smoker.

Action Your doctor will perform diagnostic tests. If he or she diagnoses cancer, treatment will depend on the type, site, and size of the tumor.

Chronic bronchitis (persistent inflammation of the airways in the lungs) may be causing your breathing problems, especially if you smoke and have had similar periods of breathlessness in the past.

Action Consult your doctor. If you smoke, he or she will tell you to stop. After performing diagnostic tests, your doctor may prescribe antibiotics. An aerosol inhaler may help relieve your breathlessness.

Pneumoconiosis (a reaction to dust in the lungs) may be causing your respiratory symptoms.

Action Consult your doctor, who will perform tests to see how badly your lungs have been affected. Your doctor may advise you to change your job. If you smoke he or she will tell you to quit because smoking will damage your lungs even more.

EMERGENCY GET MEDICAL HELP NOW!

Pulmonary embolism (a blood clot in the lung) may be causing your breathlessness, especially if you have coughed up blood-stained phlegm.

Action Your doctor will probably admit you to the hospital. If the diagnosis is confirmed, you will be treated with drugs to dissolve the blockage and to prevent additional blood clots from forming.

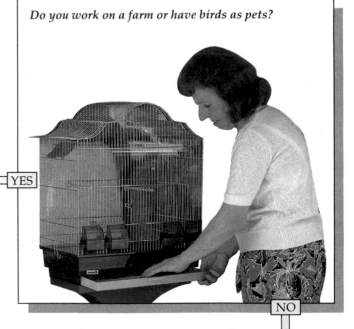

Do you work on a farm or have birds as pets?

Hypersensitivity pneumonitis (an allergic response to dusts found in some grains and in animal excretions, dander, and feathers) may be causing your breathing problems. Allergy attacks can cause breathlessness, along with coughing.

Action Consult your doctor, who will perform diagnostic tests to find out what triggers your allergic reaction. If an allergy is discovered, your doctor may advise you to change jobs or to wear a protective mask at work. Your doctor may prescribe drugs to reduce airway inflammation.

YES

NO

MONITOR YOUR SYMPTOMS
WHEEZING

If you have a chest cold, you may wheeze when you exhale. As long as your breathing is normal in other respects you should not be alarmed. Wheezing is usually audible only through a stethoscope, but it may become louder when you exhale vigorously. Loud wheezing can signal a more serious condition that requires medical attention, especially if you also feel breathless or if breathing is painful.

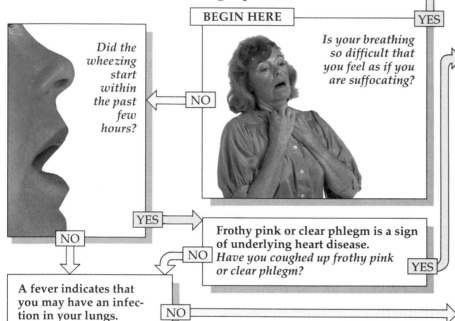

BEGIN HERE

Is your breathing so difficult that you feel as if you are suffocating?

YES

Did the wheezing start within the past few hours?

NO

NO

YES

Frothy pink or clear phlegm is a sign of underlying heart disease.
Have you coughed up frothy pink or clear phlegm?

NO

YES

**EMERGENCY
GET MEDICAL HELP NOW!**

A severe asthma attack may be causing your wheezing.

Action A prolonged asthma attack may require hospital admission. Your doctor will give you drugs to control the attack. If your breathing is severely impaired, the doctor may place you on a mechanical ventilator to help you breathe.

CALL YOUR DOCTOR NOW!

Pulmonary edema (a dangerous buildup of fluid in the lungs) from heart failure may be causing your wheezing.

Action Sit in a chair to make breathing easier. If your doctor suspects pulmonary edema, he or she may admit you to the hospital, where you will be given oxygen and drugs to treat possible heart failure. Further treatment will depend on the underlying problem.

Action Consult your doctor if you cannot make a diagnosis from this chart.

NO

A fever indicates that you may have an infection in your lungs.
Is your temperature 100°F (38°C) or higher?

NO

YES

Acute bronchitis (infection of the airways in the lungs) is a possible cause of your symptoms.

Action Take aspirin or an aspirin substitute and stay in a warm, humid environment. Drink plenty of fluids to reduce the stickiness of the mucus in your airways so it is easier to cough up. If your condition does not improve within 48 hours, call your doctor.

Persistent wheezing is a sign of a chronic lung disorder, such as asthma or chronic bronchitis (persistent inflammation of the airways in the lungs).
Do you wheeze a little almost every day, especially in the morning?

YES

NO

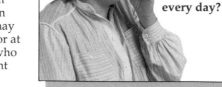

Do you cough up gray, green-yellow phlegm almost every day?

YES

A mild attack of asthma is probably making you wheeze.

Action An allergy often triggers asthma. Try to find out which substances provoke a reaction and avoid them. The cause may be substances in your home or at work. Consult your doctor, who can prescribe drugs to prevent future attacks.

Chronic bronchitis may be causing your wheezing, especially if you smoke or have had similar episodes in the past.

Action Consult your doctor. If you smoke, he or she will tell you to quit. He or she may prescribe antibiotics or give you an aerosol inhaler to help you breathe more easily.

NOISY BREATHING: STRIDOR

Noisy, high-pitched breathing that becomes worse when you inhale is known as stridor. The condition occurs when the large central airways become obstructed. In adults, common causes include a cancerous or benign tumor of the trachea (windpipe), larynx (voice box), or bronchus; swelling of the larynx from infection; or an inhaled object. In children, stridor is often caused by bacterial infection of the epiglottis (the flap of cartilage that prevents food and liquid from entering the windpipe) or an inhaled object. Stridor that starts suddenly can be terrifying for a child. Fear can cause the child to hyperventilate (breathe very rapidly or deeply), which makes the symptoms worse.

Infection of the epiglottis, restricting incoming air

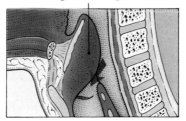

Tumor of the trachea

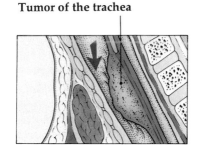

Infection and swelling of the larynx

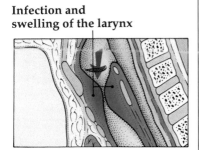

CHEST PAIN

Chest pain can be caused by conditions other than respiratory problems, including heart disease, disorders of the muscles and bones, and abdominal disorders. People who perform heavy physical labor or who exercise strenuously can also experience chest pain if they are not in good condition.

The most common cause of chest pain produced by lung disease is pleurisy (inflammation of the pleura, the membrane that surrounds the lungs). Pain occurs when the two layers of the pleura, which are usually separated by a lubricating fluid, rub together. Pleurisy may start gradually or abruptly. The pain is sharp and becomes worse when the person moves, coughs, or breathes deeply. A common cause of such pain is lung infection. A blocked blood vessel in the lung, which causes oxygen deprivation and death of the affected lung tissue, can also produce pleural pain. Pleurisy often accompanies and complicates the treatment of lung tumors, tuberculosis, and collapsed lung.

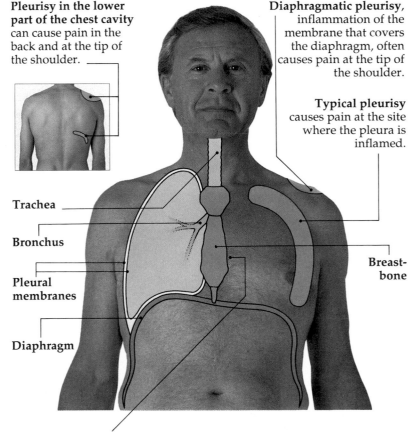

Pleurisy in the lower part of the chest cavity can cause pain in the back and at the tip of the shoulder.

Trachea

Bronchus

Pleural membranes

Diaphragm

Diaphragmatic pleurisy, inflammation of the membrane that covers the diaphragm, often causes pain at the tip of the shoulder.

Typical pleurisy causes pain at the site where the pleura is inflamed.

Breast-bone

Inflammation of the trachea or a bronchus (tracheitis or bronchitis) often causes pain behind the breastbone. It worsens with coughing but improves as the person coughs up phlegm.

■ **Sites of chest pain**
The illustration above shows the most common sites of chest pain caused by respiratory disease.

MONITOR YOUR SYMPTOMS
COUGHING

When you have a cold or allergy, or if you smoke, your throat can become irritated or partially obstructed by mucus. Coughing, which can either produce phlegm or be "dry," is your body's attempt to clear any inhaled object, congestion, or inflammation from your lungs or throat. But coughing sometimes signals a more serious respiratory tract disorder – such as emphysema, lung cancer, or heart failure – that needs medical treatment.

A cough accompanied by a high temperature and breathlessness indicates that an infection may be present in your lungs.
Is your temperature 100°F (38°C) or higher? **YES** **NO**

BEGIN HERE
Is your cough dry (without phlegm)? **NO** → *Did the cough start within the past week?* **YES** →
YES ↓
NO →

Hoarseness occurs when your vocal cords become inflamed. If you are hoarse and have a cough, you may have an upper respiratory tract infection.
Is your voice hoarse or have you recently lost your voice? **YES** →

Infection of the upper respiratory tract is possible. Both bacterial and viral infections can produce symptoms of hoarseness and coughing.

Action Stay in bed, drink plenty of fluids, and call your doctor if your condition does not improve in 24 hours. You may need to take antibiotics.

NO ↓

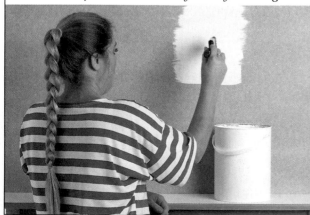

Could you have just inhaled a small piece of food, such as a peanut? **YES** →

An inhaled object in your airway could be making you cough. If you cannot cough up the object, you must have it removed.

Action Consult your doctor if the cough persists for more than an hour or if you can feel that something you inhaled is now lodged in an airway.

NO ↓

NO → *Have you had a dry cough with no other symptoms for more than a month?* **NO**
YES ↓

Could you have inhaled the fumes of an irritating substance or particles to which you may be allergic?

CONSULT YOUR DOCTOR WITHOUT DELAY!

Inflammation of an airway, from an allergy, smoking, or nonbacterial pneumonia, is probably making you cough. Your cough could also signal lung cancer, especially if you are over 40 and a smoker.

Action Your doctor will probably arrange for you to have diagnostic tests, such as a chest X-ray or bronchoscopy (see page 80).

YES →

Irritation of the airways caused by inhaling smoke or chemicals may be causing your cough.

Action If the cough does not go away within half an hour or if you become short of breath, call your doctor.

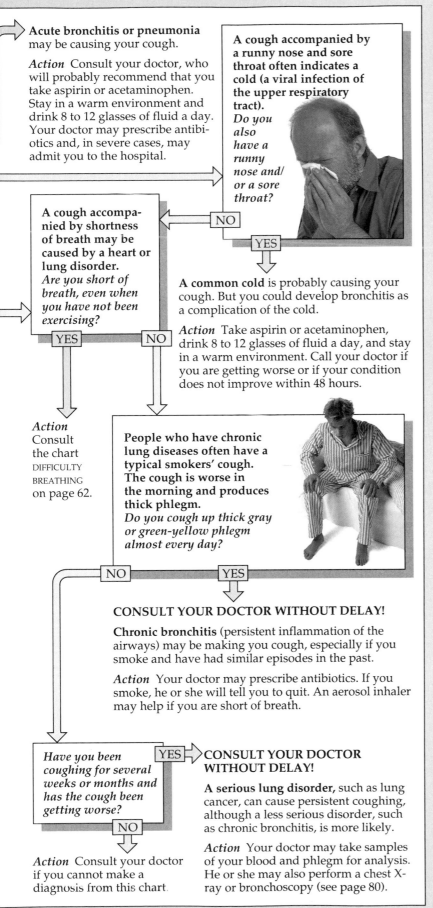

Acute bronchitis or pneumonia may be causing your cough.

Action Consult your doctor, who will probably recommend that you take aspirin or acetaminophen. Stay in a warm environment and drink 8 to 12 glasses of fluid a day. Your doctor may prescribe antibiotics and, in severe cases, may admit you to the hospital.

A cough accompanied by a runny nose and sore throat often indicates a cold (a viral infection of the upper respiratory tract).
Do you also have a runny nose and/ or a sore throat?

NO

YES

A cough accompanied by shortness of breath may be caused by a heart or lung disorder.
Are you short of breath, even when you have not been exercising?

YES   NO

A common cold is probably causing your cough. But you could develop bronchitis as a complication of the cold.

Action Take aspirin or acetaminophen, drink 8 to 12 glasses of fluid a day, and stay in a warm environment. Call your doctor if you are getting worse or if your condition does not improve within 48 hours.

Action Consult the chart DIFFICULTY BREATHING on page 62.

People who have chronic lung diseases often have a typical smokers' cough. The cough is worse in the morning and produces thick phlegm.
Do you cough up thick gray or green-yellow phlegm almost every day?

NO   YES

CONSULT YOUR DOCTOR WITHOUT DELAY!

Chronic bronchitis (persistent inflammation of the airways) may be making you cough, especially if you smoke and have had similar episodes in the past.

Action Your doctor may prescribe antibiotics. If you smoke, he or she will tell you to quit. An aerosol inhaler may help if you are short of breath.

Have you been coughing for several weeks or months and has the cough been getting worse?

YES

NO

CONSULT YOUR DOCTOR WITHOUT DELAY!

A serious lung disorder, such as lung cancer, can cause persistent coughing, although a less serious disorder, such as chronic bronchitis, is more likely.

Action Your doctor may take samples of your blood and phlegm for analysis. He or she may also perform a chest X-ray or bronchoscopy (see page 80).

Action Consult your doctor if you cannot make a diagnosis from this chart.

COUGH

Coughing is your body's normal reaction to irritation of the mucous membranes that line your airways. Coughing usually signals infection of the airways or lung tissue, which causes inflammation that irritates your airways.

Dry cough

A dry cough does not produce any phlegm. This kind of cough characterizes the early stages of acute bronchitis or pneumonia, or an acute asthma attack. When the cough is persistent, especially at night, it can be very tiring. A dry cough also occurs when a person has inhaled an object, a piece of food, or some fluid into the airways. The inhaled substance severely irritates the mucous membranes lining the person's respiratory tract. The person experiences either an explosive cough or a coughing attack in an attempt to dislodge the inhaled substance. If coughing fails to expel the object, the person may need emergency medical attention (see page 131).

Productive cough

A productive cough is one that produces phlegm. If you have a productive cough that brings up large quantities of green, yellow, brown, or black phlegm, consult your doctor promptly. Clear phlegm is usually of no concern.

The coughing up of blood-stained phlegm, called hemoptysis, can signal a serious underlying disease. A single episode that produces very little blood may not be serious and the trachea, bronchi, and lungs would still be considered healthy. But coughing up bloody phlegm repeatedly or in substantial quantities can be a sign of a lung tumor, an embolism in the lung (see page 106), tuberculosis (see page 91), acute pneumonia, or an abscess in the lung. Rust-colored phlegm suggests pneumonia. Pink, frothy phlegm occurs with pulmonary edema (see page 120) and is caused by red blood cells leaking into the fluid in the air sacs of the lung.

Plenty of fluids
Drinking plenty of water and other fluids helps to relieve the dehydration that often occurs when you have a cold or cough. Fluid consumption also helps dilute and loosen secretions in the nose and airways.

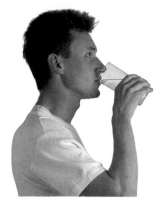

OVER-THE-COUNTER REMEDIES

When you shop for a cold remedy, you are confronted with a wide range of over-the-counter preparations for the relief of symptoms. Some remedies do relieve symptoms and most are safe if used as directed. But some do little to relieve symptoms. Others can even be harmful.

Menthol, eucalyptus, and camphor

Cough-suppressant tablets containing menthol and eucalyptus oil can relieve minor throat irritation and soothe nasal passages. Inhaling camphor ointment or oil that has been rubbed on the chest and neck may help relieve nasal congestion, but it is extremely poisonous if swallowed. Do not give children preparations that contain camphor.

Compound cough preparations

Some cough medications contain a mixture of drugs in amounts that are too low to be effective. Others combine ingredients that cancel the effects of one another, such as cough suppressants (which can cause retention of phlegm) combined with expectorants (which increase bronchial secretions). Some preparations contain antihistamines (drugs that inhibit the effects of histamine, a substance produced by certain types of white blood cells in your body, which causes watery eyes and a runny nose). They can cause drowsiness in some people.

HOW YOU CATCH AND FIGHT THE COMMON COLD

Nearly 200 different viruses can cause the common cold. Viruses are easily transmitted from one person to another by droplet transmission – when an infected person coughs or sneezes – or by touching your mouth after touching the hands of an infected person or an object that the person has touched.

1 Virus particles that enter your nose may become trapped in your nasal hairs. Chemical substances in the moist nasal linings destroy some of the particles. Other virus particles invade cells lining the back of your throat and nose.

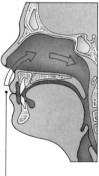

Virus particles

2 Inside your body's cells, the viruses replicate themselves. Hundreds of new virus particles are released, invade new cells, and multiply again.

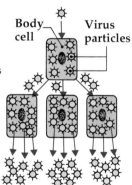

Body cell   Virus particles

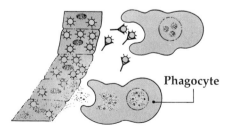

3 Your temperature rises in an attempt to eliminate the virus, producing a fever. Irritation caused by virus particles makes you sneeze, which expels some virus particles.

4 The blood supply to your infected nasal lining increases, delivering large numbers of white blood cells called lymphocytes. The blood vessels become engorged, causing the nasal lining to secrete fluid, giving you a runny nose and, later, congestion.

Infected nasal lining

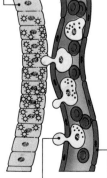

Lymphocyte   Blood vessel

5 Some of the lymphocytes produce proteins called antibodies that immobilize virus particles. Other lymphocytes secrete potent chemicals that destroy infected cells along with the virus particles inside them.

Antibody

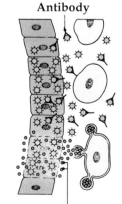

Chemicals

6 Other white blood cells called phagocytes engulf and digest immobilized virus particles, destroyed particles, and damaged cells. Within a few days your body has won the battle and you "get over" your cold.

Phagocyte

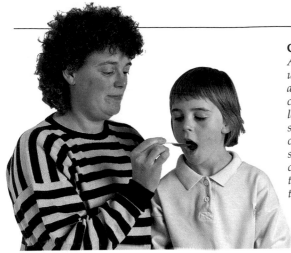

Cough syrup
A simple cough syrup usually contains sugar and coloring. Most cough syrups are harmless and can be useful in soothing irritating coughs in children. But some contain alcohol, so check the contents on the label before giving the syrup to a child.

Cough syrups

Some cough preparations contain soothing substances, such as sucrose (sugar) syrup or glycerol (a syrupy type of alcohol), and moisturizing agents designed to relieve throat irritation. Such preparations may also help loosen increased bronchial secretions during a cold.

Mucolytic medications

Manufacturers claim that mucolytic medications alter the consistency of bronchial secretions, making it easier to cough up phlegm. The evidence for this claim is weak. Some mucolytic medications may be effective, but they can cause irritation and trigger a reflex narrowing of the airways, which makes breathing difficult.

Antiseptic throat lozenges
Antiseptic throat lozenges combine a local anesthetic, which relieves soreness, and antiseptic agents, which inhibit the growth of bacteria, to help relieve the pain of sore throats.

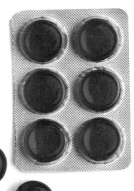

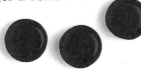

Cold and cough remedies

Aspirin and acetaminophen help relieve some symptoms of colds and coughs. They reduce fever and relieve headaches, body aches, and sore throats. Do not give aspirin to children under 16 because there is a small risk they might develop a rare disease called Reye's syndrome.

Over-the-counter cold remedies may contain a mild painkiller, such as aspirin or acetaminophen; an antihistamine; caffeine; vitamin C; and flavorings. These preparations may help relieve your cold symptoms, but they cannot "cure" your cold, which must run its course.

ASK YOUR DOCTOR
COUGH AND COLD REMEDIES

Q I have chronic bronchitis. Why did my doctor tell me not to take a cough suppressant?

A Most prescription cough-suppressant preparations contain derivatives of opium, such as codeine, that cause you to retain phlegm. This effect could cause mucus to dry and plug your lungs and airways, worsening your bronchitis. These preparations can also cause nighttime wakefulness and daytime sleepiness.

Q I recently had a severe cold and took decongestant tablets to relieve my stuffy nose. My doctor has since told me not to take these tablets because they could worsen my high blood pressure. How do these tablets work?

A These tablets reduce the secretion of mucus by narrowing blood vessels in the nose. Some nasal decongestants contain drugs that work like the natural hormone epinephrine, which raises blood pressure. Prolonged use of decongestants could raise your already high blood pressure by narrowing blood vessels and stimulating your heart.

Q Does inhaling a menthol chest rub really do any good when I have a chest cold and a cough?

A Inhaling menthol vapors does not have any medical benefit for the treatment of colds, bronchitis, or sinusitis. But some people report that, when they have a cold, the pleasant-smelling menthol vapors soothe their irritated airways. Menthol chest rubs that contain camphor are poisonous if swallowed.

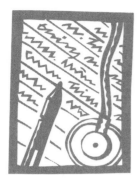

YOUR DOCTOR'S EXAMINATION

I F YOU DEVELOP respiratory symptoms, your doctor will perform a physical examination to find out the cause. If your doctor suggests a hospital examination, he or she will order several tests. But in the office, your doctor can gain useful information about your respiratory health just by observing you and using a stethoscope.

Your skin coloring
Lack of oxygen causes a bluish discoloration of the skin called cyanosis (below). The discoloration appears under the fingernails and toenails and in the person's lips, nose, and ears.

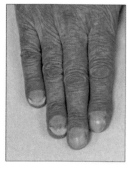

Your doctor will look for signs of respiratory difficulty as soon as you enter his or her office. Such signs reveal themselves in the way you walk, your skin coloring, or your breathing. After questioning you about your medical history, your doctor will perform a physical examination. He or she will observe, tap on, and feel your chest, and will listen to it with a stethoscope.

OBSERVING YOUR BREATHING

Your doctor will take your pulse and check your breathing rate. The normal adult breathing rate averages between 12 and 17 breaths per minute. After strenuous exercise, this rate can increase to 80 breaths per minute.

Fast breathing occurs in people who are anxious or who have an infection or an overactive thyroid gland. Drug overdoses, head injuries, and obesity induce slower-than-normal breathing rates.

Breathing patterns

The doctor will check your breathing patterns. Rapid, shallow breathing occurs in people with lung conditions such as pleurisy (see page 89), who find it painful to expand their lungs fully. Deep, irregular breathing is the body's way of compensating for an inability to exhale enough carbon dioxide. Such breathing occurs in people with kidney failure, emphysema, or uncontrolled diabetes. It may also result from an acetaminophen overdose, a head injury, liver disease, or liver failure. Stress-related hyperventilation is rapid and shallow or abnormally deep breathing that can upset the chemical balance in the blood, causing numbness and tingling in the fingers and toes and around the mouth.

The beginning of the examination
You may be asked to undress and lie on the doctor's examining table. The doctor watches your chest as you inhale and exhale to look for any chest deformity and to find out whether both your lungs expand equally.

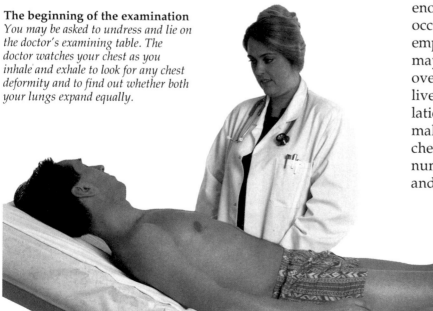

Palpating your chest
To find out whether the two sides of your diaphragm move equally when you breathe, your doctor will examine you as shown at right, placing his or her fingertips on the sides of your chest with thumbs meeting over your spine.

upright with your arms down or with your arms held forward; the doctor sits or stands behind you. The doctor may place his or her hands on your chest (close together or wide apart, depending on the area of the chest being examined).

Percussion

When the doctor taps your chest with his or her fingers, the sound produced can vary, depending on the density of the underlying lung tissue. Doctors describe the different sounds they hear as either resonant (the normal sound in most areas), hyperresonant (more resonant than normal), or dull.

When the doctor taps the chest of a person with severe emphysema, collapsed lungs, or asthma, he or she hears a hyperresonant sound because the lung tissue contains more air than normal. The doctor hears a dull chest percussion when he or she taps an area of the lung that has become dense because of pulmonary fibrosis (fibrous tissue in the lung) or because the person's pleura (the two-layered membrane that surrounds the lungs) is abnormally thick or the space between the membranes is filled with fluid. The doctor can locate normal and abnormal areas by listening to the different sounds in each area.

YOUR CHEST

Your doctor uses a technique called palpation to feel the movement of your chest while you breathe. Palpation can give your doctor clues about what might be wrong. During the procedure, you sit

Sites for percussion
Shown at right are the places on your rib cage that the doctor may tap to compare the sounds produced.

The technique of percussion
The doctor places one hand, palm down, on your chest or back, with fingers slightly separated and the middle finger firmly pressed over the area to be tapped. He or she uses the middle finger of the other hand to sharply strike the middle finger resting on your body, and listens to the quality of the sound produced.

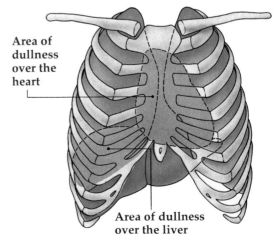

Area of dullness over the heart

Area of dullness over the liver

What your doctor listens for
Percussion of a healthy lung produces a resonant sound in all areas, except over the heart and the upper edge of the liver, where the sound is dull.

71

Vibrations

The doctor may place the sides of both hands on your chest and ask you to repeat words that resonate well, such as "ninety-nine." Your doctor can feel the vibrations made by sound waves coming from your larynx to your chest wall by way of your airways. The vibrations increase if a lung is more dense than normal. This change occurs in people with pneumonia or pulmonary fibrosis. Vibrations decrease when the pleura thickens or when fluid builds up in the pleural space.

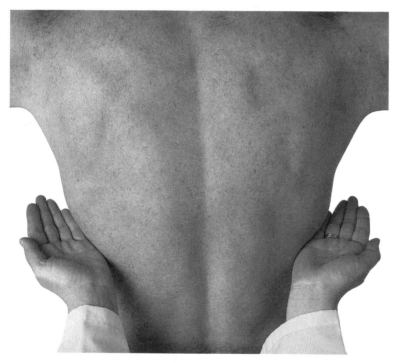

Vibrations in your chest
The doctor will ask you to say words such as "ninety-nine" so that he or she can feel the vibrations through your chest.

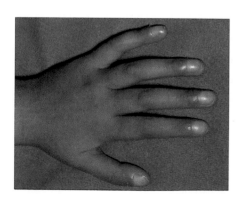

Finger clubbing
The doctor examines the tips of your fingers and toes to see if they have changed in shape. Finger clubbing (shown at left), in which the nails become more curved and the ends of the fingers become bulbous, occurs in people with lung cancer, pulmonary fibrosis, chronic bronchitis, tuberculosis, emphysema, or a lung abscess.

USING A STETHOSCOPE

The doctor uses a stethoscope to listen to the sound of your breathing. This procedure is called auscultation. Through the stethoscope, the doctor hears the sound of air passing through your trachea, bronchi, or smaller airways. The sound can vary in loudness, rhythm, and pitch.

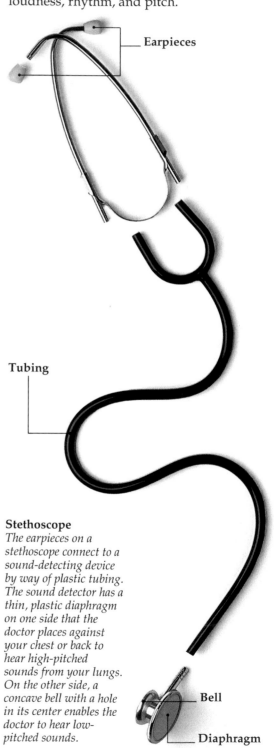

Earpieces

Tubing

Stethoscope
The earpieces on a stethoscope connect to a sound-detecting device by way of plastic tubing. The sound detector has a thin, plastic diaphragm on one side that the doctor places against your chest or back to hear high-pitched sounds from your lungs. On the other side, a concave bell with a hole in its center enables the doctor to hear low-pitched sounds.

Bell

Diaphragm

Breath sounds
The graphs at right represent the wave-forms made by sounds your doctor might hear in your lungs as you breathe.

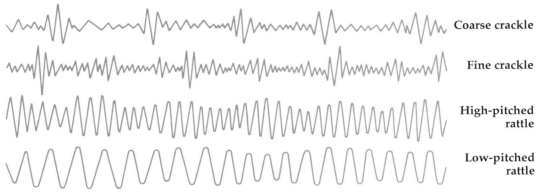

Coarse crackle

Fine crackle

High-pitched rattle

Low-pitched rattle

NORMAL BREATH SOUNDS

Vesicular breathing
This sound is the gentle rustling noise your doctor can hear in the smallest bronchi and alveoli of your lungs. The sound is loudest during inhalation but fades away rapidly when you begin to exhale.

Tracheal breathing
This sound is heard from the area along the breastbone. The sounds made when you inhale and exhale are equally loud, and a period of silence occurs between the times you inhale and exhale.

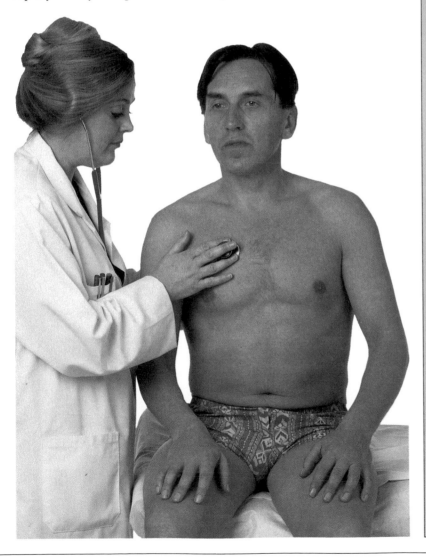

ABNORMAL BREATH SOUNDS

Bronchial breathing
This type of breathing sounds similar to tracheal breathing but occurs in areas of the lung other than those near the trachea. Bronchial breathing indicates the presence of lung disease, such as pneumonia or a collapsed lung.

Diminished breathing
The intensity of lung sounds can sometimes fall when a barrier prevents the breathing sounds from reaching the chest wall. This can happen in people with emphysema, obstruction of a bronchus, or fluid in the pleural space.

Pleural rub
If the membranes that surround the lungs become inflamed, rubbing can be heard during both inhalation and exhalation. The sound may occur in people who have pneumonia.

Crackles
These sounds are also called râles and can be heard when you inhale. They occur when the alveoli are filled with fluid. Doctors hear fine crackles in people with chronic bronchitis, emphysema, or pulmonary fibrosis. Coarse crackles, or bubbling sounds, are heard in people with chronic bronchitis or asthma who cannot cough up and spit out phlegm.

Rattles
These sounds, also called rhonchi, are either low- or high-pitched and occur when you inhale and exhale. They are heard when air passes through large airways that are narrowed by secretions, an obstruction, or muscle spasm in the bronchus. The pitch varies with the width of the opening and the speed of the airflow.

IMAGING THE LUNGS

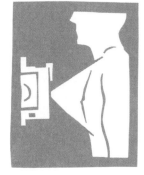

A FTER YOUR DOCTOR has questioned you about your symptoms and examined you for any abnormalities, he or she will decide whether or not to order any tests and will determine which procedures are appropriate. Imaging techniques can help your doctor diagnose many lung diseases. Doctors also frequently use these techniques as a guide when taking tissue or fluid samples.

How a chest X-ray is taken
During a chest X-ray, the technician will ask you to take and hold a deep breath, which expands your chest and lowers your diaphragm. Holding your breath enhances the quality of the X-ray image of your lungs. During the period of X-ray exposure, which usually lasts only a fraction of a second, you must remain very still; any movement produces a blurred image that is difficult for the radiologist to interpret. The procedure is safe and painless.

Doctors can examine your lungs in two ways: invasively and noninvasively. In an invasive procedure, the doctor introduces tubes, instruments, or a radioactive substance into your body. In noninvasive procedures, doctors examine your body from the outside. In general, doctors prefer to use a noninvasive method because it is safer. But sometimes doctors must use an invasive procedure.

IMAGING TECHNIQUES BASED ON X-RAYS

An X-ray is a form of invisible, electromagnetic wave radiation that is closely related to light waves but has a shorter wavelength, a higher frequency, and higher energy.

Plain chest X-ray
A plain chest X-ray is often the first test a doctor performs to investigate lung disorders. To obtain an image, the radiologist (a doctor who specializes in

The most common X-ray views
The standard X-ray view is obtained while you stand. The film is positioned in front of your chest, with the X-ray source 6 feet behind you. If you are very sick and cannot stand, a chest X-ray may be performed while you are in bed, with the X-ray source in front of you. But the resulting image usually does not help the doctor diagnose the problem as well as the X-ray obtained when you stand. Another X-ray is taken from the side. If an abnormality shows up on the front view, the side view allows the doctor to see whether the problem is located on the front or back of the chest. If the doctor is uncertain, he or she may take X-rays in other positions.

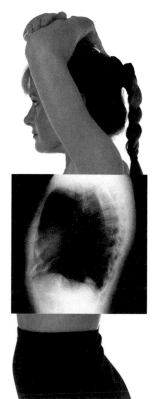

Front view

Side view

imaging techniques) passes X-rays through your chest and onto a piece of film. Dense objects, such as your ribs, absorb X-rays and appear white on the film; less dense organs, such as healthy lungs, allow X-rays to pass through easily and look dark on the film.

The presence of air in healthy lung tissue permits X-rays to travel easily through the lungs. But, when the lung's air spaces are filled with fluid, as in a person with pneumonia, the diseased tissue absorbs X-rays and appears white on the film. A malignant (cancerous) tumor often looks like a rounded, dense lump, occasionally having small white spikes of cancerous tissue that penetrate the surrounding normal tissue. Other disorders, such as fibrosis (scarred lung tissue), can appear as subtle shadowing throughout the lungs.

Employers often require chest X-rays before people begin some jobs, to screen for some infectious diseases. Taken at regular intervals, X-rays also help monitor people whose work may put them at an increased health risk. A series of chest X-rays can also gauge how quickly a lung disease is progressing.

The person's exposure to X-rays usually lasts less than a second. The amount of X-rays a person receives during a chest X-ray examination is minimal but the effects are cumulative, so the number of exposures should be limited.

Fluoroscopy

During fluoroscopy, a continuous stream of X-rays passes through the person's lungs, while the doctor views the moving image on a fluorescent screen, rather than on X-ray film. This process enables the doctor to see the lungs move.

Fluoroscopy involves longer exposure to radiation than a plain chest X-ray, so it is used much less frequently. Use of this technique is diminishing, but it can help a doctor guide a biopsy needle to the site of an abnormality when a sample of tissue or fluid is needed.

CT SCANNING

During computed tomography (CT) scanning, a moving radiation source passes narrow beams of X-rays through the person at different angles. Detectors that follow the radiation source pick up the beams and send electronic signals to a computer. The computer uses this information to produce a two-dimensional, cross-sectional image of a section of the body.

Before the scanning is performed, the person often receives an injection of a contrast medium (see page 76) that highlights blood vessels and hollow organs. CT scanning can detect small masses in the lungs, the extent of malignant lung tumors, and disease in the chest wall and lymph nodes.

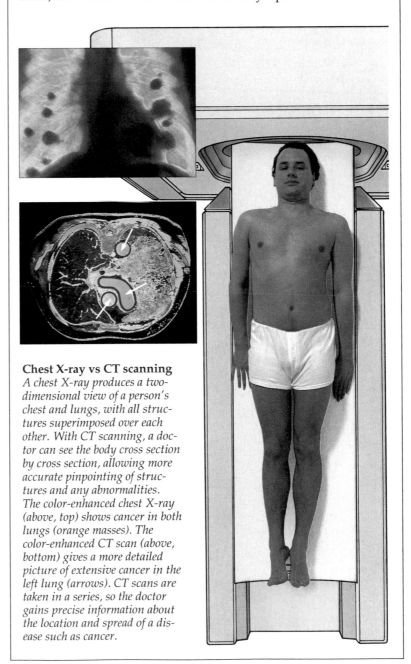

Chest X-ray vs CT scanning
A chest X-ray produces a two-dimensional view of a person's chest and lungs, with all structures superimposed over each other. With CT scanning, a doctor can see the body cross section by cross section, allowing more accurate pinpointing of structures and any abnormalities. The color-enhanced chest X-ray (above, top) shows cancer in both lungs (orange masses). The color-enhanced CT scan (above, bottom) gives a more detailed picture of extensive cancer in the left lung (arrows). CT scans are taken in a series, so the doctor gains precise information about the location and spread of a disease such as cancer.

MRI SCANNING

Magnetic resonance imaging (MRI) does not use X-rays to make an image of the body. The person lies inside a large cylindrical magnet that produces a powerful magnetic field. Pulses of radio waves are sent into the body, and the atoms in the person's body respond with radio signals. A computer converts these signals into an image. MRI is a noninvasive procedure that produces an image similar to that of a CT scan. It provides doctors with detailed, precise information about the structure of the body. The procedure takes 20 to 30 minutes and produces no known side effects.

ULTRASOUND

Ultrasound scanning is a noninvasive imaging technique that uses high-frequency sound waves emitted by a device called a transducer. The sound waves are inaudible to the human ear. The technician holds the transducer on the person's skin over the part of the body to be viewed, and the device sends sound waves into the body. The transducer, which also acts as a receiver, picks up the ultrasound waves that are reflected off the body's internal organs. A computer then transforms the reflected sound waves into an image on a screen.

Diagnostic uses

Ultrasound waves pass readily through fluid and soft tissues but are reflected by air and absorbed by bone. For this reason, the technique is most valuable for investigating fluid-filled areas. For example, it can detect fluid surrounding the lungs (pleural effusion). It also helps guide the doctor when he or she must take a sample of fluid from the lining of the lung or a sample of tissue from an abnormality at the edge of the lung. Ultrasound has no side effects.

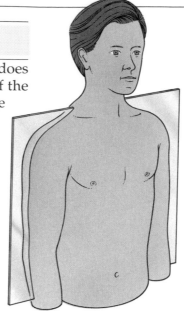
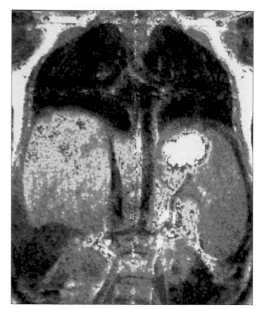

Magnetic resonance imaging
Magnetic resonance imaging (MRI) can produce cross sections of a person's body in any direction. The color-enhanced MRI scan shown above reveals a vertical section of the trunk. The healthy lungs appear as very dark areas at the top. The lungs look relatively small because the person was exhaling while the scan was taken.

RADIONUCLIDE SCANNING

X-ray techniques use an external form of radiation. But in radionuclide scanning, doctors introduce a radioactive substance called a radionuclide into the person's body. A gamma camera detects the amount and location of the gamma radiation (a type of radiation having a shorter wavelength than X-rays) given off by this substance and sends it to a computer. The computer creates an image from this information.

Gallium scanning

Before performing a gallium scan, doctors inject a radioactive form of the metal gallium into the person's bloodstream. Scanning is performed 72 hours later. Doctors study the density of the gallium in the person's lungs and compare it with the element's density in other sites in the person's body.

Gallium scans can reveal certain lung problems, such as a lung abscess, and enable doctors to study some lung dis-

WHAT IS A CONTRAST MEDIUM?

A contrast medium is a dye through which X-rays cannot pass that doctors sometimes inject into a person's bloodstream or ask the person to drink before obtaining an X-ray. If the substance is given by injection, the person may experience a flushing, warm, or hot sensation. Some contrast media contain iodine, which can produce an allergic reaction. Reactions are uncommon, but if you have had an allergic reaction to a contrast medium in the past, you should tell your doctor.

eases such as lung cancer. AIDS patients who are prone to an uncommon form of pneumonia sometimes receive these tests. Gallium scans can reveal lung disease earlier than an ordinary X-ray image. No side effects are known.

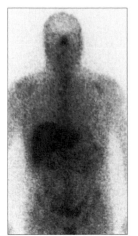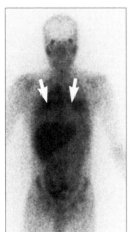

Normal   **Abnormal**

Gallium scan
The gallium scan above right shows an abnormal distribution of gallium in both lungs (arrows), revealing the extent of lung tissue affected by sarcoidosis, a disease that produces scarring of lung tissue.

PULMONARY ANGIOGRAPHY

Pulmonary angiography is performed when doctors suspect pulmonary embolism (a blood clot blocking the pulmonary artery, the blood vessel that carries blood from the heart to the lungs). This test is especially valuable if other, less invasive tests have not been conclusive.

During pulmonary angiography, the doctor inserts a tube called a catheter into a vein in the person's arm or groin and carefully guides it along the vessel until it reaches the pulmonary artery. The doctor injects a contrast medium (see page 76) through the catheter into the pulmonary artery and its branches in the person's lungs. The contrast medium outlines the arteries, which appear white on an X-ray. If an embolus is present, the artery often appears to end abruptly at the point where the clot lies.

V/Q LUNG SCANS

Doctors perform two radionuclide scans (V/Q scans) to rule out a pulmonary embolism (a blood clot in the lung). V stands for ventilation (air flow) and Q for blood flow.

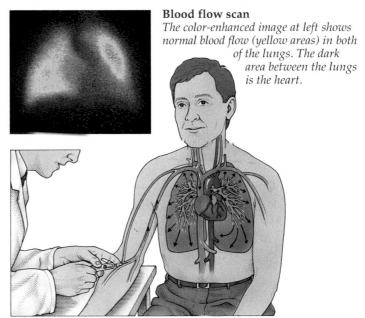

Blood flow scan
The color-enhanced image at left shows normal blood flow (yellow areas) in both of the lungs. The dark area between the lungs is the heart.

Performing a blood flow scan
The blood flow scan requires the injection of a radioactive substance into the person's bloodstream. A gamma camera detects the distribution of the radioactive substance in the body. The absence of radioactivity in a part of the lungs suggests damage in this area, either from a blood clot blocking a pulmonary artery or from lung disease.

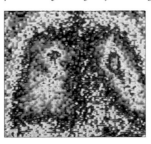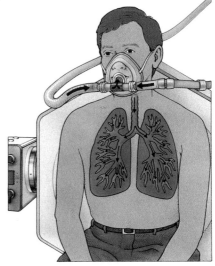

Ventilation scan
The color-enhanced scan above shows normal ventilation in both lungs. The mottled blue areas show the distribution of inhaled radioactive gas. The light area in the center is the heart.

Performing a ventilation scan
The person inhales a radioactive gas or spray, which spreads to all areas of the lungs that are ventilated. A gamma camera picks up the gamma rays emitted by the inhaled substance. If the ventilation scan is normal but blood flow to an area is absent, the diagnosis is likely to be an embolism.

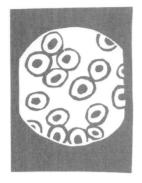

TESTS AND PROCEDURES

I MAGES OF THE LUNGS provide much useful information. But some lung diseases are not revealed on these images. For example, a chest X-ray of a person with asthma is usually normal, even though the person may experience severe difficulty breathing. This explains why doctors also use other methods of measuring how well a person's lungs are functioning.

One of the simplest methods of measuring lung function is a test called spirometry. Doctors find it extremely useful for diagnosing respiratory disease and monitoring the effect of treatment. But doctors also use other tests to rule out possible causes of breathing difficulties. If a lung disorder is diagnosed, doctors may order tests, such as bronchoscopy, to identify the cause.

SPIROMETRY

Doctors use a machine called a spirometer to measure the amount of air a person inhales and exhales over time. The spirometer provides important information about how well the person's lungs are functioning. For example, the airways of a person with asthma or chronic bronchitis are narrowed, causing reduced air flow. The spirometer can measure the airway resistance (see page 21) to the air the person exhales.

Using the spirometer
The person inhales and exhales air from a tube attached to the drum of the spirometer. A piston moves up and down as the volume of air inside the drum changes. A pen registers the process.

Respiratory measurements
The graph at right shows measurements of lung capacities.

Total lung capacity
Total lung capacity is the volume of air that a person's lungs contain when he or she takes as deep a breath as possible (maximum inhalation). This capacity is usually 5.8 liters.

Tidal volume
When a person is breathing quietly, the amount of air that moves in and out is called the tidal volume. This amount is about 0.5 liter.

Forced expiratory volume
The forced expiratory volume at 1 second (FEV_1) is the volume of air exhaled in the first second when a person exhales as hard as possible. Obstructive lung diseases, such as asthma and chronic bronchitis, reduce this volume.

Vital capacity
The vital capacity is the difference between the amount of air left in the lungs (residual volume) after a maximum exhalation and the total lung capacity. The doctor can measure this amount by having the person inhale until his or her lungs are full and then exhale as much as possible.

Residual volume
The amount of air left in the lungs after a person exhales as much as possible (maximum exhalation) is known as the residual volume. It equals about 1 liter.

Spirometer drum

Maximum inhalation

Maximum exhalation

Volume in liters

Time in seconds

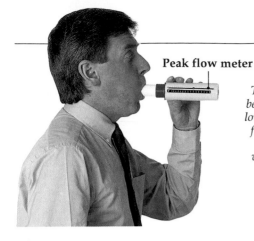

Peak flow meter

Peak flow measurements
The highest rate at which air can be exhaled, called the peak flow, is lower in people with asthma. Peak flow can be easily measured with a portable peak flow meter into which the person exhales as hard as possible. People with asthma can monitor their condition at home and report the results to their doctor.

An invader in the airways
The red specks in the photograph at right (magnified 1,200 times) are Streptococcus pneumoniae *bacteria, found in a phlegm sample from a person with bacterial pneumonia.*

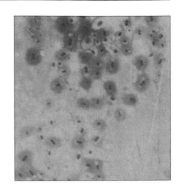

DIFFUSION CAPACITY TEST

Diffusion is the process by which a substance passes from an area of higher concentration to one of lower concentration. A diffusion capacity test measures how easily gases such as oxygen and carbon dioxide can diffuse between the bloodstream and the air sacs of the lungs. The ability of these gases to diffuse can be reduced in diseases that decrease the surface area of the lungs' air sacs or by the loss of surrounding capillaries, thickening of the tissue between the air sacs and capillaries, or anemia.

1 The doctor introduces a small, measured amount of carbon monoxide into the air that the person inhales from a spirometer.

2 Most of this gas passes into the person's bloodstream by diffusion.

Red blood cell

Capillary

Blood flow

Carbon monoxide

Inhaled air plus carbon monoxide

Alveolus

Exhaled air plus carbon monoxide

Spirometer

3 The doctor measures the level of carbon monoxide in exhaled air.

4 The doctor can calculate how well gases can pass from the lungs into the bloodstream by subtracting the amount of carbon monoxide left in the exhaled air from the amount administered in the inhaled air.

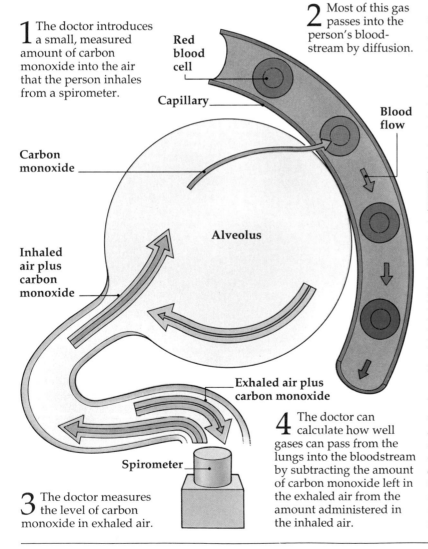

PHLEGM SAMPLES

If you have an infection or inhale an irritant, such as cigarette smoke, your airways produce more mucus. The excess mucus induces coughing, which forcibly expels the mucus from your airway into your mouth as phlegm.

A laboratory technician can stain a sample of phlegm and examine it under a microscope, or place it in a dish containing nutrients that encourage the growth of bacteria. If you have an infection, the type of bacteria that has caused the infection will grow. These procedures help your doctor identify the microorganism causing a lung infection. Cancerous cells in phlegm indicate lung cancer.

TESTING THE BLOOD

Doctors sometimes order blood tests to help diagnose a respiratory problem. Such tests analyze a sample of the person's blood to detect the numbers of red and white blood cells (see below), levels of hemoglobin (see page 30), or the presence of bacteria or antibodies (proteins produced by your body that fight invading microorganisms).

What blood samples can show
A reduced number of red blood cells in the blood can indicate a form of anemia. A bacterial lung infection may increase the numbers of some types of white blood cells in the blood.

White blood cells

Red blood cells

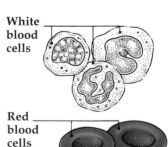

Tests of blood gases

Doctors can test the severity of a lung disease and monitor the effects of treatment by measuring the amounts of oxygen and carbon dioxide in blood drawn from an artery in the person's wrist, forearm, or groin. Analyzing the blood shows how well the blood is absorbing oxygen and excreting carbon dioxide.

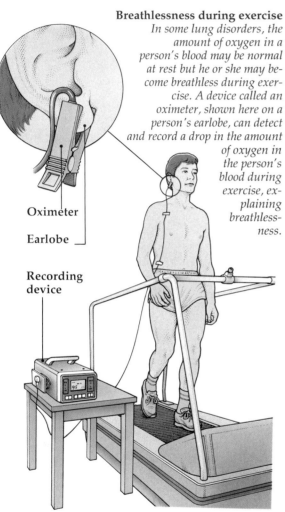

Breathlessness during exercise
In some lung disorders, the amount of oxygen in a person's blood may be normal at rest but he or she may become breathless during exercise. A device called an oximeter, shown here on a person's earlobe, can detect and record a drop in the amount of oxygen in the person's blood during exercise, explaining breathlessness.

Oximeter

Earlobe

Recording device

Oximetry

An oximeter is a small device that can be attached to a person's earlobe (see above) or fingertip to detect the amount of oxygen in the person's blood. Oximetry is less accurate than sampling blood from a person's artery, but it is simple and painless, and it can measure oxygen levels over time. For example, an oximeter can monitor blood oxygen levels while a person is sleeping.

ENDOSCOPY

An endoscope is a long, flexible instrument that the doctor can insert through an opening in the body, such as the mouth, or through an incision. The endoscope, which is capable of transmitting light, allows the doctor to view internal structures. The forms of endoscopy that help doctors examine the lungs and chest include bronchoscopy, thoracoscopy, and mediastinoscopy (see page 81).

These procedures enable the doctor to examine the lungs and airways for signs of disease and to take small samples of tissue (biopsy specimens) from the airway walls or the lungs. The samples can be examined for cancer or infection.

HOW IS BRONCHOSCOPY PERFORMED?

1 The person is sedated and given a local anesthetic to numb the throat, voice box, and trachea (windpipe). The doctor inserts the bronchoscope into the person's mouth and passes it to the back of the throat. This process enables the doctor to view the vocal cords.

Bronchoscope

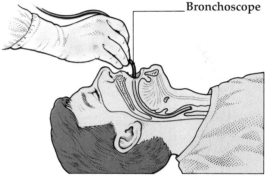

2 The doctor passes the tube farther down the trachea and into the bronchi (see right). The doctor can now inspect the person's airways for disease and take small samples of tissue or collect secretions by suction.

Bronchi

VIEW THROUGH BRONCHOSCOPE

3 A laboratory worker stains and inspects samples under a microscope or cultures them to find out what microorganisms may be causing the disorder.

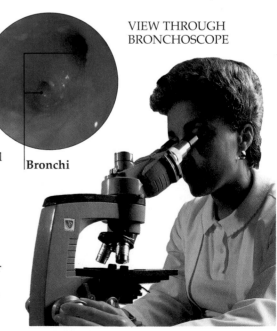

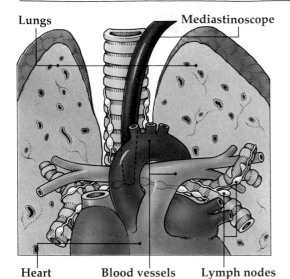

Lungs **Mediastinoscope**

Heart **Blood vessels** **Lymph nodes**

Mediastinoscopy
With the person under general anesthesia, the surgeon makes an incision in the chest wall and investigates areas near the heart and large blood vessels using a type of endoscope called a mediastinoscope. Doctors often perform this procedure to take samples of tissue, such as lymph node tissue, from areas inside the mediastinum (the central compartment of the chest, between the lungs). Sometimes these areas are hard to reach.

During thoracoscopy, the doctor uses a type of endoscope called a thoracoscope to inspect the pleura (the membrane covering the lungs) through a small incision in the side of the person's chest.

PLEURAL AND LUNG BIOPSIES

Fluid often collects between the layers of a diseased pleura, the membranous sac covering the lungs. Doctors call this condition pleural effusion. The fluid compresses the lungs, sometimes causing the person to become breathless. The doctor may take samples of pleural fluid (see below) and of pleural tissue (a pleural biopsy) for examination. The doctor examines these samples under a microscope to look for cancerous cells or for any signs that indicate infection.

To diagnose some lung diseases, a surgeon may take samples of lung tissue (lung biopsy) by opening the chest while the person is under general anesthesia. Examining the biopsy tissue often provides information important for diagnosis.

Sampling pleural fluid and tissue
After cleaning and anesthetizing the area, the doctor inserts a needle attached to a syringe into the pleural space to withdraw fluid. Infection or inflammation makes the fluid look cloudy or bloody. The doctor may also take a sample of pleural tissue (pleural biopsy specimen) to help identify the cause of the fluid accumulation.

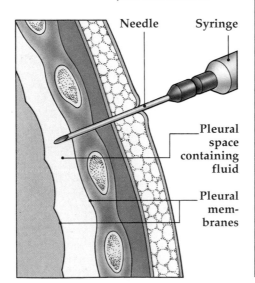

Needle **Syringe**

Pleural space containing fluid

Pleural membranes

ASK YOUR DOCTOR
TESTS AND PROCEDURES

Q My 7-year-old son often has an asthma attack when we visit his grandparents' farm. Is a test available to find out what triggers these attacks?

A Your son may be allergic to something on the farm, such as ragweed pollen, house-dust mites, or cat or dog dander (skin flakes). Your doctor can give your son a skin test in which a small amount of the suspected allergen will be introduced into his skin. Anything to which your son is allergic will produce a reaction on his skin, revealing the allergens your son should avoid.

Q My wife has pneumonia and must have a series of blood tests over the next few weeks. Why are so many tests needed?

A In some forms of pneumonia, the microorganism causing the infection is difficult to identify. Your wife's immune system will produce proteins, called antibodies, that fight these organisms. By analyzing blood samples taken over time, her doctor can detect the rising level of antibodies and identify the organism causing your wife's pneumonia.

Q My doctor is going to examine my lungs with a bronchoscope to try to find out the cause of a recurrent lung infection. Will I have to stay in the hospital?

A No. During bronchoscopy, a flexible tube will be inserted down your throat and into your airways while you are sedated. The procedure takes less than 30 minutes. After you awaken, a friend or family member can take you home.

CHAPTER FOUR

LUNG DISEASES AND DISORDERS

A WIDE RANGE OF diseases and disorders can affect your lungs. Doctors often classify these disorders three ways: disorders characterized by inflammation (caused by infections or allergies and other autoimmune disorders); cancers and other growths; and inherited disorders. But some conditions that affect the lungs cannot be categorized easily. For example, doctors once viewed asthma as an inherited allergic disorder. But doctors now think it may be an acquired inflammatory condition.

Substances that are present in the air you breathe can cause many lung diseases. But these substances are rarely harmful to people with healthy lungs. Serious lung infections develop mainly when a person has an underlying lung problem caused by asthma, smoking, or poor nutrition. Emphysema, cancer of the lungs and bronchus, and chronic bronchitis can be caused by inhaled cigarette smoke. Occupational lung diseases, such as coal workers' pneumoconiosis, are caused by inhaling tiny particles of coal dust or other minerals in large quantities. In some lung diseases, the lungs become scarred for no known reason. Other diseases that affect the lungs, such as cystic fibrosis, are inherited.

Problems can also arise when the circulation in your lungs does not function properly. For example, large blood clots called emboli can lodge in a lung's blood vessels, preventing blood from reaching the tiny air sacs called alveoli where the blood exchanges oxygen and carbon dioxide. A condition called pulmonary hypertension may be caused by an underlying disorder or may occur for no known reason. Pressure builds up in the blood vessels that carry blood to the lungs. The heart must work harder to pump blood through the lungs but eventually may not be able to keep up with its task. If this happens, the person soon experiences breathlessness because the amount of oxygen reaching his or her blood has been reduced.

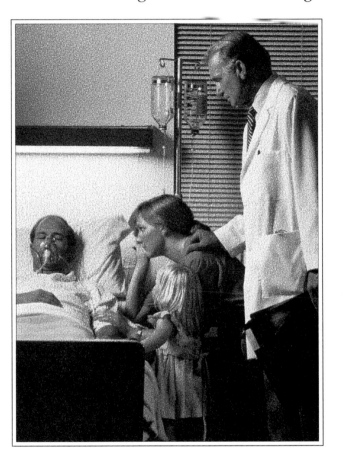

Obstruction of an airway is life-threatening and requires emergency treatment. Airways can become blocked when a person accidentally inhales an object or when the lungs fail to inflate following an injury. In a premature baby, breathing difficulty from lack of surfactant (a substance that prevents the air sacs in the lungs from collapsing) can also be life-threatening.

The incidence of some lung diseases could be reduced by limiting exposure to cigarette smoke and industrial dusts. Vaccines can help protect people against some lung diseases. Other disorders, such as bronchitis, respond well if detected and treated early.

LUNG INFECTIONS

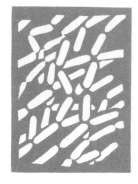

MICROORGANISMS POPULATE the air you breathe. When someone sneezes, thousands of disease-carrying organisms are projected into the air. These organisms can enter your lungs and airways when you inhale. Bacteria, viruses, and fungi can infect your lungs, causing pneumonia (inflammation of the lungs) and other serious lung infections.

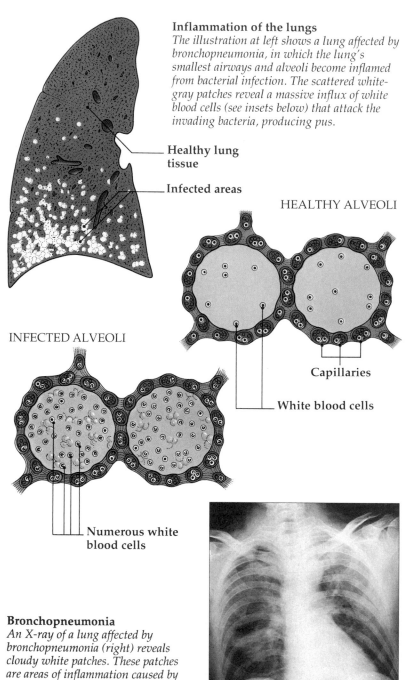

Inflammation of the lungs
The illustration at left shows a lung affected by bronchopneumonia, in which the lung's smallest airways and alveoli become inflamed from bacterial infection. The scattered white-gray patches reveal a massive influx of white blood cells (see insets below) that attack the invading bacteria, producing pus.

Healthy lung tissue

Infected areas

HEALTHY ALVEOLI

INFECTED ALVEOLI

Capillaries

White blood cells

Numerous white blood cells

Bronchopneumonia
An X-ray of a lung affected by bronchopneumonia (right) reveals cloudy white patches. These patches are areas of inflammation caused by bacterial infection.

Disease-producing organisms affect not only the tissues of the lung but also structures such as the double-layered membrane that covers the lungs (pleura) or the linings of the airways. Infants, older people, and people with weakened immune systems are especially susceptible to respiratory infections.

BACTERIAL PNEUMONIA

A variety of bacteria can produce pneumonia. The most common cause of bacterial pneumonia in adults is the organism *Streptococcus pneumoniae*. Men contract pneumonia two to three times more often than women. Symptoms include loss of appetite, fever, sweating, violent shivering, joint and muscle pain, and headache. Coughing, breathlessness, and chest pain soon follow. The pain often gets worse when the person breathes deeply. People who have pneumonia usually produce green or yellow phlegm that sometimes contains blood.

The doctor attempts to identify the cause from the results of blood and phlegm tests and prescribes antibiotics. In mild cases, the person may not have to be hospitalized and usually recovers after about 7 days. More serious cases require hospitalization. If tests show a low level of oxygen in blood taken from an artery, the doctor may give the person extra oxygen. People with severe pneumonia may need several weeks or months to completely recover.

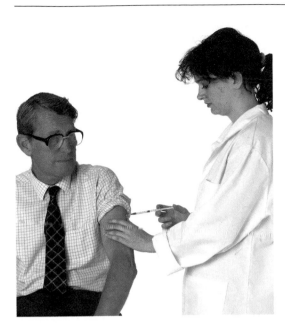

Lifesaving flu shots
Bacterial pneumonia can develop after a case of influenza. For this reason, doctors recommend yearly influenza vaccinations for older people and for people with chronic kidney, lung, or heart diseases. Doctors also recommend them for health care workers who care for patients at risk of contracting influenza.

MYCOPLASMAL PNEUMONIA

Mycoplasmal pneumonia is relatively common in people between the ages of 5 and 25 but is less common in people older than 65. Accounting for about 50 percent of pneumonia cases, it often occurs as an epidemic in people living together in close quarters, such as military recruits. A tiny penicillin-resistant organism, *Mycoplasma pneumoniae*, causes this type of pneumonia.

In mild cases, the person may just feel "under the weather" and can remain out of bed and active. For this reason, the disease is sometimes called "walking pneumonia." In addition to respiratory symptoms of coughing and breathlessness, the person may develop a rash, a headache, neck stiffness, and joint inflammation. Antibiotics help clear up this type of pneumonia. Recovery takes about a week.

Spreading pneumonia
The organism that causes mycoplasmal pneumonia is transmitted from one person to another by inhaling droplets expelled in a sneeze or a cough. Transmission often occurs when people are in close contact, such as in families, schools, and dormitories.

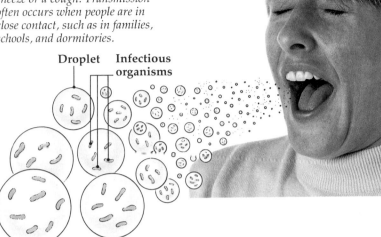

Droplet   Infectious organisms

ASPIRATION PNEUMONIA

Aspiration pneumonia occurs when vomit or food is inadvertently inhaled into the lungs. This sometimes happens when a person is unconscious (see below). It can also occur if a person has difficulty swallowing, sometimes as a result of a neurological illness such as a stroke, or as a result of a condition affecting the esophagus (which extends from the throat to the stomach). Bacteria in the inhaled matter infect the lungs. The doctor may admit the person to the hospital to treat the condition that caused the person to inhale the infected matter, especially if the person has a severe reaction. Doctors treat aspiration pneumonia with antibiotics.

LUNG ABSCESS

A lung abscess is an infected cavity in the lung that is filled with pus and dead tissue. It occurs relatively rarely but can develop after accidentally inhaling food or secretions from the mouth and throat. A lung abscess can also occur after bacterial pneumonia or when a lung tumor obstructs a bronchus.

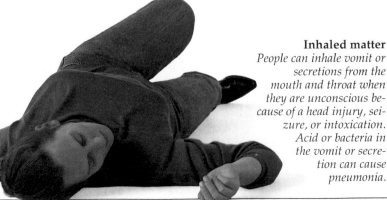

Inhaled matter
People can inhale vomit or secretions from the mouth and throat when they are unconscious because of a head injury, seizure, or intoxication. Acid or bacteria in the vomit or secretion can cause pneumonia.

Q FEVER

Q fever is an uncommon infection first seen in 1935 when it spread among slaughterhouse workers in Australia. The organism responsible for Q fever, *Coxiella burnetii*, infects sheep, goats, and cows in rural areas. The animals excrete it in feces, milk, and urine. The organism can survive for

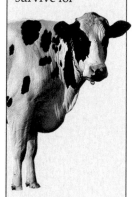

months in soil, straw, machinery, and clothing. People become infected predominantly by inhaling contaminated material. Q fever is actually two distinct illnesses, one affecting the person's heart and the other affecting the lungs and liver. Symptoms of lung infection include a dry cough and chest pain. Doctors treat Q fever with an antibiotic drug to which *Coxiella burnetii* is sensitive. The illness is often so severe that affected people must enter the hospital. The disease usually clears up within 2 weeks.

LEGIONNAIRES' DISEASE

Scientists first described the rare bacterial condition known as legionnaires' disease in 1976 – after an epidemic of severe pneumonia broke out among veterans at an American Legion convention in Philadelphia. Although the bacterium that causes the disease is found in virtually all water supplies, it thrives in large, water-cooled air-conditioning systems and accumulates in plumbing systems where water stagnates, for example in shower heads. Legionnaires' disease is three times more common in men than in women and has its highest incidence in those aged 40 to 70, especially if they are smokers, diabetics, alcoholics, and people taking drugs that suppress the immune system.

Symptoms appear suddenly, within a week of infection. High fever, chills, and muscle aches are followed by a cough that produces small amounts of clear phlegm. Severe headaches, confusion, diarrhea, and abdominal pain can occur.

A person suspected of having legionnaires' disease will probably be admitted to the hospital. The doctor usually starts treatment with intravenous antibiotics, such as erythromycin. Younger people usually recover fully from the disease, but elderly or unhealthy people can die of lung damage.

What causes actinomycosis?

The bacterium that causes actinomycosis, Actinomyces israelii *(seen below, magnified 16,000 times), lives in the mouth and throat and in dental plaque. The bacterium causes a lung infection when a person inhales it.*

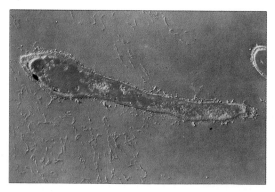

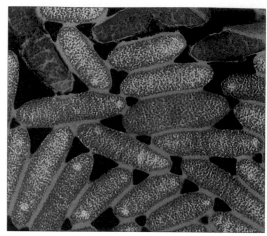

Cause of legionnaires' disease
The bacterium Legionella pneumophila *(shown in the color-enhanced photograph above, magnified 13,000 times) causes legionnaires' disease.*

ACTINOMYCOSIS

This very rare bacterial infection can affect a person's lungs, abdomen, or neck. Actinomycosis of the lungs causes severe inflammation and may produce irreversible damage to lung tissue.

Symptoms include recurrent mild fever, weight loss, coughing, and phlegm production. The phlegm may be discolored and/or streaked with blood. Pus can collect in the pleural space, a condition known as empyema. Abscesses that form in the neck may rupture and drain through the skin. Doctors treat the person with high doses of intravenous (given through a vein) penicillin for 4 weeks. The person must take penicillin tablets for another 6 months.

VIRAL PNEUMONIA

Viral pneumonia, which accounts for 10 to 15 percent of all pneumonias, is spread by inhaling droplets expelled in an infected person's sneeze or cough. After 1 or 2 days, the person experiences a sudden high fever, violent shivering, muscle aches, and a headache, followed by breathlessness and coughing.

The doctor may prescribe antibiotic drugs, even though antibiotics are effective only against bacteria, until a firm diagnosis of viral pneumonia is made. The doctor performs blood tests the first time a person visits the office, and again a month later. These tests usually identify the virus that caused the infection. The doctor may treat a person with a mild case of viral pneumonia at home.

OPPORTUNISTIC PNEUMONIAS

Opportunistic pneumonias occur when bacteria, viruses, or fungi infect people whose immune systems are already impaired. Such people include those who are receiving drug treatment (such as chemotherapy) that suppresses the immune system and people with acquired immune deficiency syndrome (AIDS). Symptoms include fever, a dry cough, and breathlessness. To identify the disease-causing organism, the doctor may perform bronchoscopy (see page 80) and may take samples of the person's bronchial secretions, blood, and tissue for examination under a microscope.

Hospitalization for pneumonia
People with pneumonia caused by the chickenpox, herpes simplex, or Epstein-Barr virus are usually admitted to the hospital.

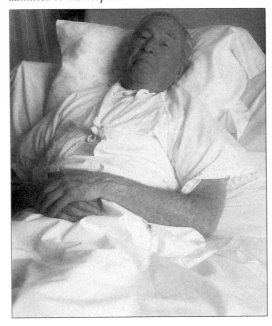

Only mild cases do not require hospital treatment. Doctors may treat the person for several weeks with drugs that kill the organism responsible for the pneumonia. Corticosteroids (drugs that fight inflammation) may be used in some cases.

EMPYEMA

Empyema is the accumulation of pus in the space between the membranes of the pleura. The most common cause is an unhealed bacterial pneumonia that spreads to and infects the pleural space. The person may experience persistent fever and chest pain. To reach a diagnosis, the doctor uses imaging techniques and withdraws pus from the pleural space for examination. Treatment includes pleural drainage through a chest tube and antibiotics. In some cases, surgery may be needed because there may be trapped areas of pus that cannot be drained completely with a chest tube.

INSERTING A CHEST DRAIN

A chest drain is a plastic tube that doctors use to remove air that has entered the space between the membranes of the pleura (which surround the lungs) and has compressed the lung. They also use a chest drain to remove fluid, blood, or pus from the pleural space.

3 Both the tube and the skin opening are wrapped with sterile gauze and saturated with iodine. The doctor tapes the tube securely to the person's chest wall. Finally, the doctor connects the tube to a suction device.

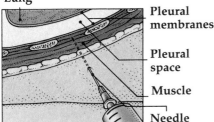

Lung · Pleural membranes · Pleural space · Muscle · Needle

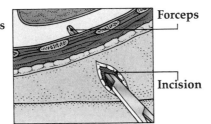

Forceps · Incision

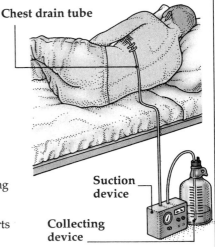

Chest drain tube · Suction device · Collecting device

1 The person lies on his or her back, while the doctor inserts a needle into the side of the person's chest, through the muscles as far as the pleura, to inject a local anesthetic.

2 The doctor makes an incision in the person's skin and dissects the underlying muscle layers. The doctor inserts a pair of forceps into the pleural space and forms a hole for the chest tube. Then he or she inserts the tube into the pleural space.

CASE HISTORY
BLOOD-STAINED PHLEGM AND FEVER

ONE SATURDAY AFTERNOON, **Marty was eating some peanuts at a baseball game. During an exciting moment, he jumped up to shout at a player. Suddenly he started coughing badly. He felt as if something was lodged in his throat. He became red-faced and breathless, but he soon recovered. Two weeks later, Marty developed a high fever and a persistent cough so he decided to visit his doctor.**

PERSONAL DETAILS
Name Marty Coolidge
Age 19
Occupation College student
Family Parents are in good health. Sister has asthma.

MEDICAL BACKGROUND
Marty has always been healthy and has rarely needed to see a doctor. He had his impacted wisdom teeth extracted 3 months ago.

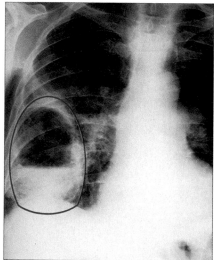

Chest X-ray
X-rays of Marty's chest reveal an abnormal area in his right lung (outlined in red, above), indicating the presence of a lung abscess.

THE CONSULTATION
Marty explains that he has not been feeling well, but he became especially concerned when he coughed up blood-streaked, green phlegm.

Removing the object
The doctor passes a flexible viewing tube, called a bronchoscope, through Marty's nose and down into the bronchi in his right lung. When the doctor sees the peanut, he grasps it with tiny forceps inserted through the bronchoscope and removes it.

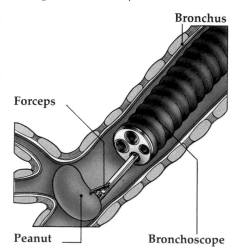

Bronchus

Forceps

Peanut

Bronchoscope

He also tells his doctor that he has lost weight and has a sharp pain in his side when he inhales deeply. The doctor asks Marty about recent events that could have caused his symptoms, and Marty recalls the choking episode during the baseball game. The doctor examines Marty and finds that his breathing is labored and shallow and that his heart rate is faster than normal. When the doctor listens to Marty's chest, he hears a rough rubbing sound coming from the right lung. The doctor arranges for Marty to have a chest X-ray and for a sample of his phlegm to be sent to the laboratory for examination. Marty's X-ray shows an abnormal white area in his right lung, and the laboratory tests show evidence of infection.

THE DIAGNOSIS
From Marty's history and the test results, the doctor diagnoses a LUNG ABSCESS caused by inhaling a peanut. The doctor explains to Marty that the peanut is lodged in and has obstructed a small bronchus (airway), which has caused the infection of tissue in his right lung. A small area of tissue has been destroyed, forming an abscess, a cavity containing pus. Infection has spread to the pleural membranes that surround his lungs. Marty's chest hurts because the inflamed and infected membranes are rubbing together. The doctor decides to admit Marty to the hospital for treatment.

THE TREATMENT
Marty is taken to the bronchoscopy room in the hospital where the doctor removes the peanut, using a bronchoscope. The doctor gives Marty a course of antibiotics to treat the remaining infection. Marty recovers fully and returns to school within a month.

PLEURAL EFFUSION

Pleural effusion is the accumulation of fluid in the space between the two layers of the pleura (see right). There are many causes of pleural effusion, including tuberculosis. Symptoms can include breathlessness, coughing, and sharp chest pain that worsens with deep inhalation. The doctor may withdraw a sample of pleural fluid and examine it to identify the organism causing the accumulation. Effusions may need to be drained through a needle or a chest drain (see page 87).

Infections of the pleura
The pleura is a double-layered membrane that covers the lungs. The two membranes are slightly separated by the pleural space, which normally contains a small amount of lubricating fluid. Infection can cause inflammation of the pleural membranes (pleurisy) or accumulation of fluid (pleural effusion) or pus (empyema) in the pleural space.

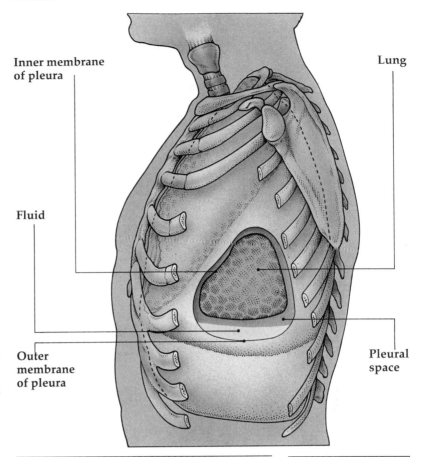

Inner membrane of pleura

Lung

Fluid

Outer membrane of pleura

Pleural space

Aspergilloma
In people with existing lung disease (such as previous tuberculosis infection or an unhealed lung abscess, which can cause a cavity to develop in the lung), inhalation of Aspergillus spores can cause the formation of a fungal ball called an aspergilloma. Aspergillomas rarely cause symptoms and may disappear without treatment. If the person repeatedly coughs up blood, the doctor may recommend surgical removal of the fungal ball.

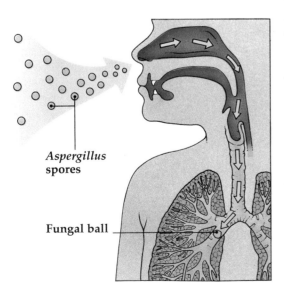

Aspergillus spores

Fungal ball

ASPERGILLOSIS

Aspergillosis is a lung disease that a person can contract by inhaling spores of *Aspergillus* fungi. Disease-causing species of *Aspergillus* are common in the environment but usually cause illness only in people with weakened immune systems. The disease takes three forms: allergic bronchopulmonary aspergillosis, aspergilloma (see left), and invasive aspergillosis. In people with allergic bronchopulmonary aspergillosis, inhaled *Aspergillus* spores trigger an asthmatic reaction. Doctors treat the asthmatic symptoms. Invasive aspergillosis is a rare but serious form of aspergillosis. Widespread fungal infection occurs throughout the lungs. It can occur in people with diseases that suppress the immune system or a chronic illness, such as diabetes. The person may have symptoms of pneumonia that do not respond to antibiotic treatment. Traditionally,

PLEURISY

Pleurisy, inflammation of the pleural membranes (see above), usually results from an inflammation of the lung, such as occurs in pneumonia or tuberculosis. It can also happen after a person has chest surgery. Normally, the two membranes, which are lubricated by fluid, slide over each other when the lungs and chest cavity expand and contract as you breathe. But if you have pleurisy, the inflamed membranes rub against each other, producing sharp chest pain that worsens each time you inhale deeply.

doctors have treated the disease with intravenous amphotericin B, an antifungal agent. Newer drugs, such as itraconazole, cause far fewer side effects than amphotericin B. Invasive aspergillosis is frequently fatal.

HISTOPLASMOSIS

Histoplasmosis is a fungal infection caused by inhalation of the fungus *Histoplasma capsulatum*, found in soil that has been contaminated by bird droppings. The affected person usually experiences only mild coughing, cold symptoms, and chest and joint pain. The body's immune system can usually fight the infection off within 10 to 14 days. When the illness persists, doctors usually prescribe antifungal drugs. A few people develop chronic (long-term) histoplasmosis infection that resembles chronic tuberculosis. But in some people the disease may spread throughout the body and ultimately be fatal.

Where does histoplasmosis occur?
The fungus that causes histoplasmosis prefers moist environments. The infection occurs in South America and the Far East; in the US, it occurs predominantly in the Ohio and the Mississippi river valleys.

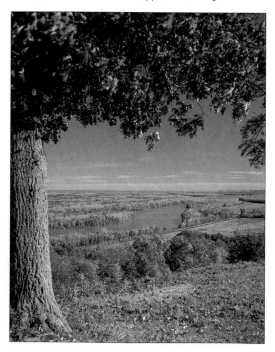

CHILDHOOD LUNG INFECTIONS

Babies and children under 5 years old are especially vulnerable to certain types of respiratory infections, which can be very severe and can require hospital admission.

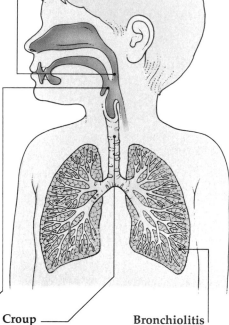

Whooping cough
This bacterial infection (also called pertussis) commonly occurs in children who have not been immunized. The child first develops a cold with a runny nose, a dry cough, and a mild fever. The cough becomes more pronounced and prolonged, ending in a "whoop." Most children can be treated at home, but the illness may last up to 10 weeks. The child should be kept warm, and antibiotics may help. Childhood immunization prevents this disease.

Epiglottitis
Epiglottitis is a rare, life-threatening bacterial infection caused by *Haemophilus influenzae*, type b. It inflames and causes rapid swelling of the epiglottis, the flap of tissue at the back of the throat that closes off the trachea when you swallow. The condition, which usually affects young children, requires emergency hospitalization, immediate placement of a tube in the trachea to keep the airways open, and antibiotics. Childhood immunization prevents the disease.

Croup
In children with croup, infection by a virus causes inflammation of the voice box, trachea, and bronchi. It is most common in children between 3 months and 5 years. Boys are more frequently affected than girls. Early symptoms include inflammation of the outer membrane of the eye and a runny nose. A fever and a cough resembling a seal's bark then develop. Symptoms typically occur at night. Doctors use humidified air and acetaminophen to treat the disorder.

Bronchiolitis
Sudden, severe bronchiolitis caused by a viral infection is common in infants but can also occur in toddlers. A virus that causes only a minor infection in an adult can cause severe bronchiolitis in an infant, so infants should be kept away from people with colds. Babies with bronchiolitis develop a fever and may refuse to eat. They may have difficulty breathing and a cough. Severely affected babies need hospital treatment with humidified oxygen and, occasionally, artificial ventilation.

TUBERCULOSIS

In the US, more than 1 million people are presently infected with tuberculosis. During the last 6 to 7 years, the incidence of reported new cases has increased.

Initial infection usually occurs during childhood and cannot be distinguished from other short-lived respiratory tract infections. In healthy people, it rarely causes symptoms. Evidence of exposure may only be obvious from a chest X-ray or a positive skin test. The organism enters the lungs when the person inhales an infectious droplet. The person's natural defense system controls the infection by restricting it to a small area in the lung. This shows up on an X-ray as a small scar. Immunity usually develops within 2 weeks to 3 months and shows up on a skin test.

The organism can lie dormant for years. Later, it can be reactivated and spread within the lungs or to other body tissues. Symptoms can include coughing, fever, phlegm production, breathlessness, night sweats, and weight loss. Affected people need prolonged treatment, sometimes with three or four drugs, but they can be completely cured.

Who is at risk?
Tuberculosis is a common infection in certain groups of people, including recent immigrants with poor nutrition, the homeless, alcoholics, undernourished people, nursing home patients, prison inmates, older people, and people with weakened immune systems.

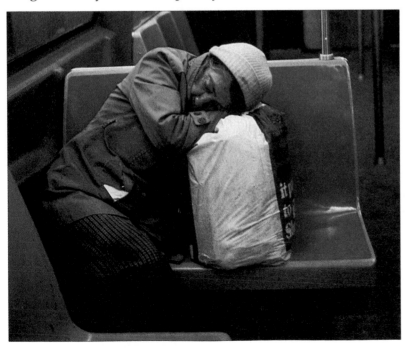

ASK YOUR DOCTOR
LUNG INFECTIONS

Q **My wife's doctor has just told her she has bacterial pneumonia. I am taking care of her at home and I need to find a babysitter for our two young children. How long will my wife need to fully recover?**

A If your wife has pneumonia with no complications that responds to treatment, her fever and cough should subside and she should begin to feel better within 5 to 10 days. But she will probably not be able to return to her normal activities for about 4 to 6 weeks.

Q **My teenage son, who has epilepsy, got aspiration pneumonia because he inhaled vomit during a recent seizure. How can I prevent this from happening again?**

A It is important that your son's seizures be as well controlled as possible. Work with his doctor to find the right dose of anticonvulsant drugs. When he does have a seizure, it is important that family and friends know how to position him correctly while he recovers, so that if he has vomited he does not aspirate (inhale) any of the vomit.

Q **My daughter's college roommate has just been diagnosed with tuberculosis. Should my daughter be examined?**

A Yes, since they have been living together. Ask the school's health service to perform a skin test that will show evidence of exposure or call your doctor. Your daughter may also need a chest X-ray, depending on the results of the skin test. If the tests show that your daughter is infected, your doctor can treat her successfully with several drugs.

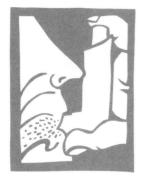

ASTHMA

I N PEOPLE WITH ASTHMA, the airways in the lungs periodically constrict, causing such frightening symptoms as breathlessness, wheezing, a sensation of chest tightness, and coughing. About 10 million Americans have asthma, and its incidence is increasing, especially among children and teenagers. Of even more concern is the sharp rise in deaths from asthma in the last 10 years.

Symptoms of asthma
Asthma symptoms, which include wheezing, breathlessness, chest tightness, and coughing, vary from day to day. During a severe asthma attack, the person's breathing becomes increasingly difficult and the heartbeat becomes rapid. The person begins sweating and experiences extreme anxiety.

Wheezing is a whistling sound the person makes when breathing. Sometimes the wheezing is so loud that it can be easily heard and sometimes it can be heard only when a doctor uses a stethoscope.

Coughing occurs from time to time and may awaken the person from sleep. The cough either can be dry or can produce small amounts of white or pale yellow phlegm.

Breathlessness is the sensation of not getting enough air, sometimes accompanied by a sensation of tightness in the chest.

Chest tightness is a sensation of pressure or constriction in the front of the chest.

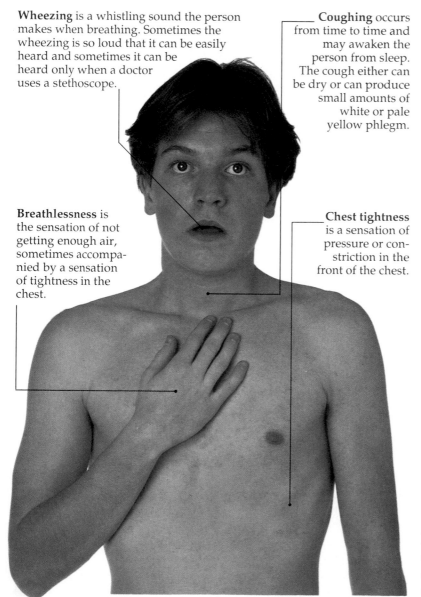

The smaller bronchi and the smallest airways, called bronchioles, in the lungs of a person who has asthma are overly sensitive and tend to become inflamed and narrowed (see BRONCHOCONSTRICTION: AIRWAY NARROWING IN ASTHMA on page 93). This narrowing makes breathing difficult. Many factors – including inhaling allergens (substances to which a person is allergic), exercising in cold weather, infection, and exposure to cigarette smoke and other airway irritants – can trigger or intensify attacks (see TRIGGERS OF ASTHMA ATTACKS on page 94). Acute asthma attacks can be fatal.

TYPES OF ASTHMA

Scientists have identified two types of asthma – allergic and intrinsic. Exposure to an inhaled allergen, such as pollen, dog or cat dander, or house-dust mites, triggers the allergic type of asthma. People with this type usually have a personal or family history of other allergic reactions, such as eczema or hay fever. This type of asthma most often starts during childhood. Intrinsic asthma does not appear to be caused by allergy; the cause remains unknown. Asthma that first occurs in adulthood is most often intrinsic. Many people who have asthma do not clearly fit into either category.

Prevalence
In the US, about 7 to 10 percent of children have asthma. Five percent of adults also have the disease. Boys develop the condition more commonly than girls,

BRONCHOCONSTRICTION: AIRWAY NARROWING IN ASTHMA

Many factors can cause the walls of the small bronchi and bronchioles of people with asthma to become inflamed. The inflammation causes a number of changes (see below). All contribute to airway narrowing. Doctors have offered several theories to explain why the airways become inflamed. These theories implicate inflammatory substances, such as histamine, released by cells in the person's lungs in response to inhaled allergens, irritant chemicals, or infectious agents.

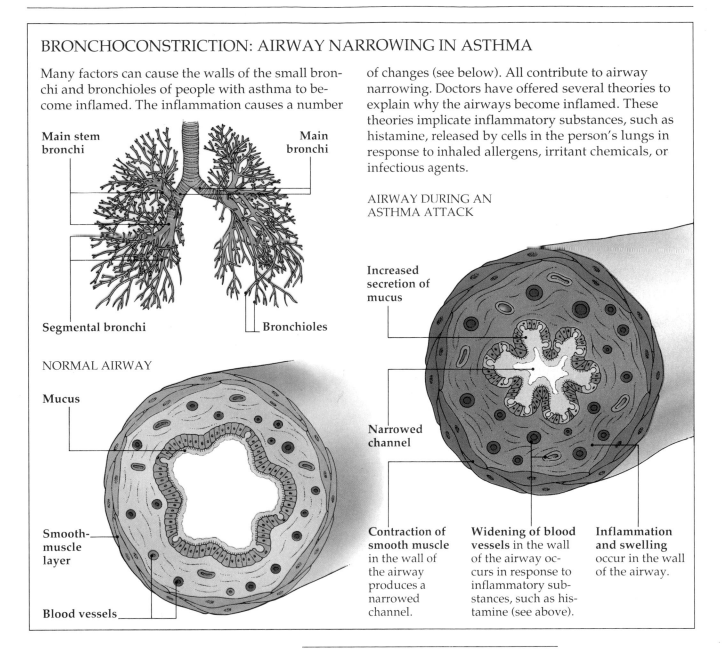

Main stem bronchi

Main bronchi

Segmental bronchi

Bronchioles

NORMAL AIRWAY

Mucus

Smooth-muscle layer

Blood vessels

AIRWAY DURING AN ASTHMA ATTACK

Increased secretion of mucus

Narrowed channel

Contraction of smooth muscle in the wall of the airway produces a narrowed channel.

Widening of blood vessels in the wall of the airway occurs in response to inflammatory substances, such as histamine (see above).

Inflammation and swelling occur in the wall of the airway.

but in adulthood, both sexes are equally affected by asthma.

Asthma is becoming more common in developed countries. Scientists have proposed various theories to explain this trend, focusing on increased air pollution, a higher number of allergens in the environment, and a greater number of synthetic chemicals to which we are exposed both at home and at work. But none of these theories has been proven. Another possible explanation for the increased prevalence of asthma is better awareness, diagnosis, and reporting.

DIAGNOSIS

The results of a physical examination and chest X-rays are usually normal between asthma attacks. A test called the FEV_1 (forced expiratory volume in 1 second) test, which measures how much air the person can exhale in 1 second, may help confirm the diagnosis. Another measurement, the peak expiratory flow rate (see page 94), checks the maximum speed at which air can flow out of the lungs. During an attack, airflow slows markedly. Between attacks, it is normal.

TRIGGERS OF ASTHMA ATTACKS

The following factors can trigger or intensify an asthma attack in susceptible people.

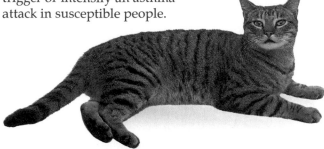

◆ Some air pollutants, such as ozone, sulfur dioxide, or diesel fuel exhaust

◆ Stress or anxiety

◆ Some drugs, such as beta blockers

◆ Vigorous exercise during cold weather, especially in children

◆ Short-term respiratory infections, such as the common cold or influenza

◆ Smoking or exposure to other people's cigarette, pipe, or cigar smoke

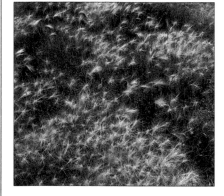

◆ Exposure to allergens, such as grass pollen (see left), house-dust mites, cat and dog dander, fungal spores, and the dust from dead cockroach bodies

◆ Exposure to substances at work

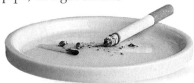

◆ Certain foods, such as eggs, or food additives, such as sulfites (in a few people with asthma)

Peak flow readings

The peak flow meter (shown at left) is a simple device. After taking a deep breath, the person exhales into it as hard as possible. The instrument measures the highest speed at which air can flow out of the person's lungs. Doctors find peak flow readings to be the most useful guide to the severity of a person's asthma. The doctor may ask the person to keep records of peak flow measurements made a number of times daily for several weeks.

Chart of peak flow

In people with asthma, charts of peak flow readings often show great daily fluctuation, with the lowest rates of airflow in the morning (called "early morning dips"). For a person undergoing treatment, early morning dips and nighttime waking indicate inadequate control of the disorder. The person may need additional medication.

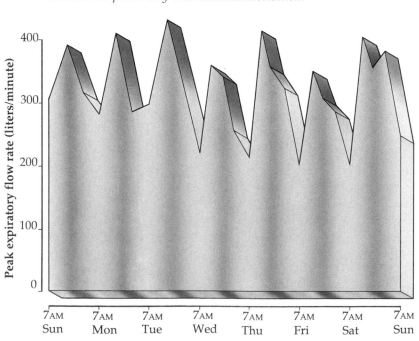

Skin tests

Skin tests can help doctors diagnose asthma because asthma is more likely to be present when the person also has a skin allergy. The most useful test is the skin prick test (shown at right).

Another way doctors diagnose an allergy is by measuring blood levels of antibodies the person's body produces when he or she has been exposed to an allergen. In one test, for example, doctors take a sample of the person's blood and add to it allergens that have been "tagged" with different substances so they can be identified later. These allergens bind to the antibodies present in the person's blood, enabling doctors to find out how much antibody is present.

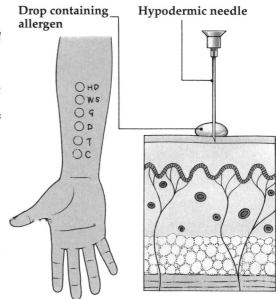

Skin prick test
The doctor places a drop containing the suspected allergen on the person's forearm, and pricks the person's skin through the drop with the tip of a small hypodermic needle. If a welt develops within 15 minutes, the test result is positive. The doctor can perform simultaneous tests for several different allergens (as shown at right). The letters on the person's arm label the different allergens. For example, HD means house-dust mite and G means grass pollen.

Drop containing allergen

Hypodermic needle

MANAGEMENT OF ASTHMA

The symptoms and severity of asthma vary enormously among affected people, so doctors must tailor treatment to a person's individual needs. The goal of treatment is to help the person lead a normal life, so that he or she can sleep through the night and even participate in exercise and sports. Self-help groups can help the person and his or her family understand the disease. See page 96 for a discussion of the medications doctors prescribe for asthma.

Preventing attacks

If you have asthma, you can prevent or minimize the occurrence of attacks by avoiding factors that trigger them. Do not smoke, and stay away from people who do. Avoid occupations with a high exposure to dust or contact with allergens. Consider giving away pets with fur or feathers or ask another family member to brush cats and dogs outdoors. Do not allow pets to sleep in your bedroom. Use synthetic instead of feather pillows. Regular vacuuming and damp dusting will reduce the number of house-dust mites in your home.

Avoid foods or food additives that are known to trigger asthma attacks. Menstruation, drugs (especially beta blockers), and physical activity may also trigger constriction of your airways. Aspirin and aspirin-containing drugs can cause asthma, especially in people who have nasal polyps (grapelike protrusions in the lining of the nose). No evidence exists that negative ion generators (ionizers) reduce the frequency of asthma attacks.

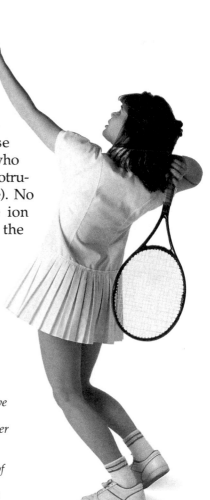

Exercise and asthma
People with asthma should stay as active as possible, and doctors encourage exercise. If you have asthma and discover that exercise triggers your symptoms, you may find it helpful to use your inhaler before you exercise. A number of professional and amateur athletes perform exceptionally well even though they have asthma.

TREATING ASTHMA WITH DRUGS

Doctors prescribe a number of drugs that can prevent or treat asthma effectively. Each person with asthma needs a drug regimen specifically tailored to his or her individual needs. Most drugs doctors use to treat asthma are known as bronchodilators. They work by relaxing the smooth muscles in the walls of the bronchi, which have become constricted, and by counteracting inflammation in the smaller airways.

RESPIRATORY TRACT INFECTIONS

If you have asthma and develop a respiratory tract infection (with a cough and phlegm), you are at increased risk of a dangerous asthma attack. Your doctor may give you antibiotics to limit the infection, if it is caused by bacteria. He or she may also prescribe corticosteroid drugs, to be taken for a few days only. The dosage will have a very specific schedule, starting with a high dose that tapers down to a low dose or to none at all. The inhaled drugs you take can also be increased. You may want to discuss an emergency plan with your doctor to help prevent a severe attack and a trip to a hospital emergency department.

WARNING

Corticosteroid drugs should never be discontinued abruptly, without a doctor's order. Stopping usage suddenly can cause the adrenal glands to stop functioning during times of stress, sending the person into shock.

DRUG GROUP	EXAMPLES	ACTION	COMMENT
BRONCHODILATORS			
Sympatho-mimetic drugs	Albuterol, isoproterenol, pirbuterol, terbutaline	When inhaled, these drugs rapidly relax bronchial smooth muscle and diminish the release of inflammatory substances.	Sympathomimetic drugs have effects on the heart and circulation, including an increased pulse, palpitations, and tremor. But these side effects are rarely troublesome.
Anticholinergic drugs	Ipratropium	This drug also relaxes bronchial smooth muscle.	Ipratropium is slower acting than sympathomimetic drugs. It takes an hour to reach its maximum effect, but the effect lasts longer.
Xanthines	Aminophylline, theophylline	The way these drugs work is uncertain. They probably interfere with the chemicals that cause bronchial smooth muscle to tighten, so these muscles can relax.	The most commonly used xanthine is a tablet form of theophylline that the person takes twice daily. The tablet releases its drug over time. Care must be taken to ensure that overdosage does not occur; theophylline is toxic at only slightly higher doses than those required to produce a therapeutic effect.
MAST CELL STABILIZERS	Cromolyn sodium	This drug helps prevent constriction of the bronchi, especially that induced by exercise or inhaled allergens. It seems to act by inhibiting the release of inflammatory substances.	Although cromolyn sodium has proven most effective in treating children and people with exercise-induced asthma, doctors do not limit its use to these two groups. It should be taken regularly as a preventive drug, especially 1 hour before exercise or exposure to known allergens.
CORTICOSTEROIDS	Prednisone, beclomethasone, flunisolide, dexamethasone	Corticosteroid drugs are powerful anti-inflammatory agents. This property makes them effective in treating asthma.	Taken in tablet form, these drugs can cause a number of unwanted side effects, such as acne, facial reddening, fluid retention, muscle weakness, and peptic ulcer. Doctors prefer inhaled corticosteroid drugs, such as beclomethasone, because they are minimally absorbed into the bloodstream and therefore have few side effects. It may take a week or longer for the drugs to achieve their maximum effect. If large quantities of corticosteroid drugs are needed, they are usually taken by mouth.

HOW TO USE AN INHALER

The fastest-acting antiasthma drugs are inhaled. If you have asthma, you should know how to use your inhaler correctly. Read the package insert and ask your doctor for advice. If you find it hard to squeeze the device while inhaling, try using a reservoir device (see below). One bronchodilator, albuterol, is available in a dry powder inhaler (see below).

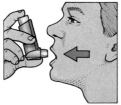

1 Shake the canister gently and remove the protective cap.

2 Exhale fully and place the mouthpiece inside your lips with your mouth open wide and your head tilted slightly backward. Do not close your lips around the mouthpiece.

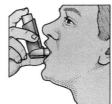

3 At the beginning of your next deep breath, depress the inhaler to release a puff. Inhale deeply and hold your breath for 10 seconds. Repeat this action a few minutes later if your doctor has prescribed more than one puff.

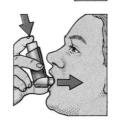

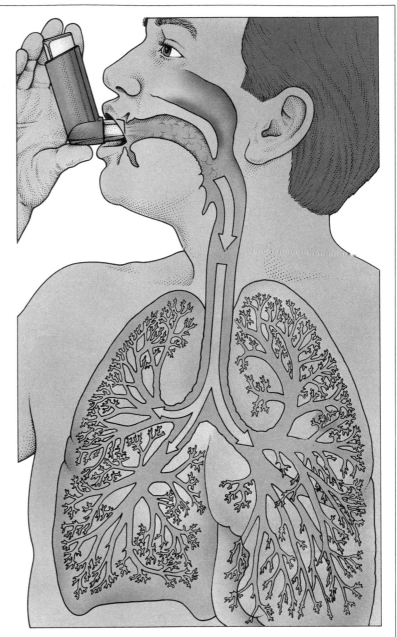

Nebulizer

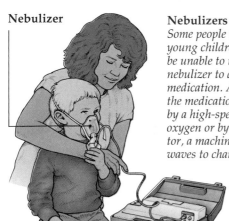

Nebulizers
Some people with severe asthma, young children, and people who may be unable to use an inhaler use a nebulizer to deliver antiasthma medication. A nebulizer disperses the medication as a fine mist, either by a high-speed stream of air or oxygen or by an ultrasonic oscillator, a machine that uses sound waves to change a liquid into a mist.

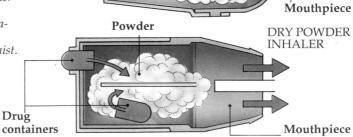

Canister

Reservoir

RESERVOIR DEVICE

Mouthpiece

Powder

DRY POWDER INHALER

Drug containers

Mouthpiece

ASK YOUR DOCTOR
ASTHMA

Q My 6-year-old daughter has been diagnosed with asthma. Will she eventually outgrow it?

A Asthma is more common in children than in adults, and there is a good chance that your daughter's asthma will clear up by the time she becomes a teenager.

Q My 17-year-old daughter is studying for her college entrance exams. She has been hospitalized twice in the last 4 months with severe asthma attacks. I am concerned that these attacks are caused by stress. What can she do?

A Asthma is seldom caused by stress alone, but stress can certainly make asthma worse. Your daughter should have skin tests. If the doctor identifies specific allergens that trigger her attacks, help her try to avoid them. Her doctor will also determine whether she needs other treatment. She must always have a supply of her medication with her. If she has another severe attack, reassure her until help arrives or until you get her to the hospital.

Q I have had mild asthma for 2 years and use an inhaler only occasionally. We don't have any pets at home, but I have recently started waking up at 4 AM feeling breathless. Why is this happening?

A For unknown reasons, people with asthma have symptoms more often in the early morning. You probably need more medication to treat the inflammation and narrowing of your airways. See your doctor. He or she may also advise you to buy a peak flow meter (see page 94) to monitor your asthma.

ACUTE SEVERE ASTHMA

Acute severe asthma is a sudden, serious attack of wheezing and breathlessness that the person's usual medication cannot control. The person may be too breathless to speak. Wheezing often diminishes as the attack worsens. The person may experience physical exhaustion and oxygen deprivation as his or her lung function deteriorates. Acute severe asthma can be fatal. The person needs immediate medical attention in a hospital emergency department.

In the emergency department, the doctor will inject a drug into a muscle or vein to open the constricted airways. He or she will also obtain chest X-rays and perform blood tests to find out the cause of the acute attack. Measuring the amounts of oxygen, carbon dioxide, and theophylline (see page 96) in the person's blood will help determine treatment. After several hours, the person may recover enough to go home. Otherwise, hospitalization will be necessary. In severe cases, the person may need help from a machine to breathe.

What to do during a severe attack
A severe asthma attack is a medical emergency. If you are with a person with asthma who is having extreme difficulty breathing, take the person to the closest hospital emergency department, dial 911, or call your local emergency medical services team. Keep the person sitting up and comfort him or her until you reach the hospital or help arrives.

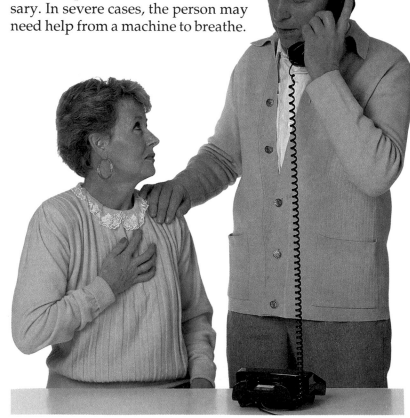

CASE HISTORY
AN ACUTE ASTHMA ATTACK

K IM HAS ASTHMA. She has had positive skin test reactions to house-dust mites, animal fur, animal dander, and other allergens. She and her family have limited her exposure to these allergens, but Kim still has fairly frequent asthma attacks that are gradually becoming more severe. Early one morning, she awakens breathless and wheezing, with a dry cough.

PERSONAL DETAILS
Name Kim Malinowski
Age 9
Occupation Student
Family Kim's family has a history of eczema, hay fever, and asthma.

MEDICAL BACKGROUND
Kim started to have minor asthma attacks at the age of 3. These attacks have gradually become more severe.

THE ASTHMA ATTACK
During the asthma attack, Kim's mother tells her to use her inhaler. Kim tries it but finds that it does not help. She tells her mother that she has tightness in her chest and her breathing becomes increasingly difficult. She begins sweating and becomes very frightened and anxious. She can inhale rapidly but wheezes loudly when she exhales. The skin around her lips becomes blue-purple, and her face becomes pale and clammy. Kim's mother becomes alarmed and drives her to the hospital emergency department.

AT THE HOSPITAL
The emergency room doctor immediately gives Kim intravenous injections of a corticosteroid drug; the bronchodilator aminophylline (see page 96) through an inhaler; and oxygen delivered through a mask.

After an hour or two, her condition improves dramatically, and she can breathe easily without oxygen. The doctor admits Kim to the hospital.

Perfecting the technique
During the discussion, the doctor explains to Kim that she needs to inhale more slowly from her inhaler and to hold her breath longer after an inhalation.

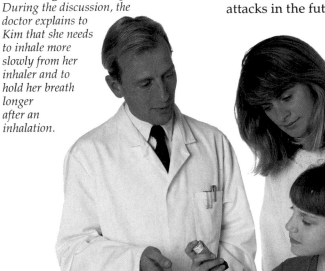

THE CONSULTATION
The next morning, the emergency room doctor talks with Kim's mother. He tells her that Kim has apparently not been using her inhaler properly. He explains that Kim must use her inhaler at the first sign of breathing difficulty, instead of waiting until an attack becomes severe. The doctor also says that if Kim's attacks are becoming more frequent even though she is using her inhaler more often, she needs to see her doctor so that he can modify Kim's treatment immediately.

The doctor then describes to Kim and her mother how to use an inhaler step by step. After the doctor is satisfied that both Kim and her mother understand the instructions, he allows Kim to go home.

THE OUTCOME
Kim becomes an expert on using her inhaler. She feels less frightened that an attack will occur and is confident that she can avoid severe asthma attacks in the future.

CHRONIC BRONCHITIS AND EMPHYSEMA

SMOKING CAUSES not only lung cancer but also chronic bronchitis and emphysema. Together, these latter two diseases are known as chronic obstructive pulmonary disease, which severely disrupts the flow of air into and out of the lungs. Smoking accounted for about 85 percent of the estimated 60,000 deaths from chronic obstructive pulmonary disease that occurred in the US in 1983.

Bronchitis is inflammation of the mucous membranes and deeper tissues of the bronchi. Acute bronchitis starts suddenly and, if limited in duration, does not cause permanent damage.

Chronic bronchitis occurs as a result of repeated infection of the bronchi and is characterized by persistent coughing up of phlegm. Emphysema causes the normal structure of the alveoli (air sacs in the lungs) to break down. They then coalesce to form larger sacs. This process reduces the surface area available for the exchange of oxygen and carbon dioxide in the alveoli and causes a reduction in the amount of oxygen in the blood.

ACUTE BRONCHITIS

Acute bronchitis often occurs when a person has an upper respiratory tract infection, such as a common cold. It can also be a complication of measles or influenza. Acute bronchitis is often mild and is usually caused by a respiratory virus. Invasion by bacteria, such as *Streptococcus pneumoniae* or *Haemophilus influenzae*, may follow and complicate the initial virus infection.

Symptoms and treatment

The symptoms of acute bronchitis include a phlegm-producing cough, a mild fever, and, in some people, slight wheezing. The doctor may diagnose acute bronchitis from the person's medical history and an examination, without further investigation. If the cough produces green or yellow phlegm, the doctor will prescribe antibiotics. Most people feel better after a few days.

What is acute bronchitis?
Acute bronchitis is inflammation of the linings of the large and medium bronchi. The inflammation stimulates the glands in the walls of the bronchi to produce abundant mucus.

Normal bronchus (cross section)

Acute bronchitis

Bronchi

Inflammation

Excess mucus

Bronchioles (smallest airways)

Limiting the infection
Cilia (fine hairs) lining the airways transport mucus upward, preventing infection from reaching lung tissue. But in children, older people, or people with a lung disease, the infection often spreads to and inflames the smallest airways or the lung tissue.

CHRONIC BRONCHITIS

Cigarette smoking is the primary cause of chronic bronchitis. Smokers compound their risk of the disease if they live in an industrial area or in a location with high atmospheric humidity or heavy rainfall. In the US, experts estimate that half of all middle-aged men who smoke 25 or more cigarettes per day will develop chronic bronchitis. The only treatment for chronic bronchitis is to quit smoking. Even symptoms present for years usually disappear within a few weeks after the smoker quits.

Symptoms

People with chronic bronchitis persistently cough up phlegm, typically when they wake and after the first cigarette of the day. Many smokers minimize this serious symptom by perceiving their cough as a normal consequence of smoking – a "smokers' cough."

People with chronic bronchitis occasionally wheeze and experience a gradual decline in their tolerance of exercise. They become progressively more breathless until they cannot walk more than a few steps without inhaling oxygen from a container they must carry with them.

LUNG DAMAGE IN NONSMOKERS

Passive smoke causes measurable changes in the lungs of healthy adults. Research shows that non-smokers exposed to passive smoke sustain as much lung damage as smokers who do not inhale or as people who smoke one to 10 cigarettes a day.

HOW DOES CHRONIC BRONCHITIS DEVELOP?

Chronic bronchitis, brought on by prolonged exposure to inhaled irritants such as tobacco smoke, causes the lining of the bronchi to produce increased amounts of mucus. It also causes structural changes in the walls of the bronchi.

Healthy bronchi
A layer of mucus, produced by glands in your bronchial walls and by goblet cells in the lining, covers healthy bronchi. The mucus traps inhaled particles, and small hairlike protrusions called cilia continuously move the mucous layer upward so you can swallow it or cough it up.

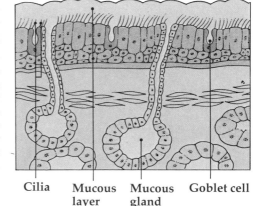

Cilia **Mucous layer** **Mucous gland** **Goblet cell**

1 Irritation of the airway lining by cigarette smoke causes increased mucus production. With persistent irritation, the mucous glands and goblet cells increase in number and size, causing a further increase in mucus production. Cigarette smoke also damages the cilia and reduces their ability to move the mucus along the airway.

2 When the cilia can no longer move the excess mucus, it stays in the airways. The retained mucus encourages the growth of bacteria, which causes repeated episodes of acute inflammation.

3 Eventually, the bronchial lining becomes so damaged that the cilia are completely destroyed.

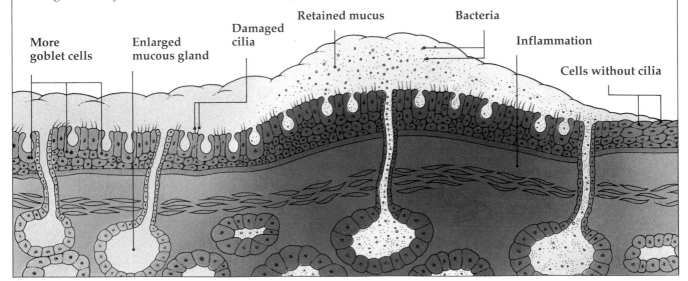

More goblet cells   **Enlarged mucous gland**   **Damaged cilia**   **Retained mucus**   **Bacteria**   **Inflammation**   **Cells without cilia**

ALPHA₁-ANTITRYPSIN DEFICIENCY

Some people inherit a deficiency of the enzyme alpha₁-antitrypsin, which protects the air sacs in the lungs. They have a higher risk of developing emphysema, even if they do not smoke. If they do smoke, the risk escalates. Alpha₁-antitrypsin can be injected intravenously for people who have the hereditary deficiency.

EMPHYSEMA

Emphysema causes a permanent change in the structure of the air sacs in the lung (alveoli), where the exchange of oxygen and carbon dioxide takes place (see below). Smoking commonly causes emphysema, but in rare cases emphysema may also arise from a hereditary deficiency of an enzyme called alpha₁-antitrypsin. Other factors that contribute to the development of emphysema include atmospheric pollution, recurrent respiratory tract infections, and respiratory tract allergies.

Signs and symptoms

At first, a person with emphysema becomes breathless only during exertion. But breathlessness eventually occurs during simple tasks, such as taking a shower. The person often coughs up phlegm if he or she also has chronic bronchitis, but coughing may be absent in later stages. Most people with emphysema also lose weight because the lack of oxygen accelerates the death of body tissue, which cannot be fully replaced. When a doctor listens to the chest of a person with emphysema, the breath sounds are very quiet and distant.

How does smoking cause emphysema?

Tobacco smoke inflames lung tissue. The inflammation attracts certain types of white blood cells that contain an enzyme destructive to the walls of the air sacs. Normally, another enzyme called alpha₁-antitrypsin inhibits this process. Tobacco smoke inactivates alpha₁-antitrypsin, allowing the destruction to proceed.

HOW DOES EMPHYSEMA DEVELOP?

Tobacco smoke provokes the release of chemicals that damage and break down the walls of the alveoli. The alveoli merge to form fewer, larger sacs. This process reduces the surface area needed for the exchange of oxygen and carbon dioxide in the lungs. Eventually, the level of oxygen in the person's blood begins to fall, leading to breathlessness and pulmonary hypertension (elevated blood pressure in the pulmonary artery) or cor pulmonale (enlargement of the right side of the heart).

Lung tissue destruction
The lung tissue at far right shows serious damage from emphysema. Destruction of the walls of the alveoli has caused the air spaces to widen, in the same way a balloon inflates.

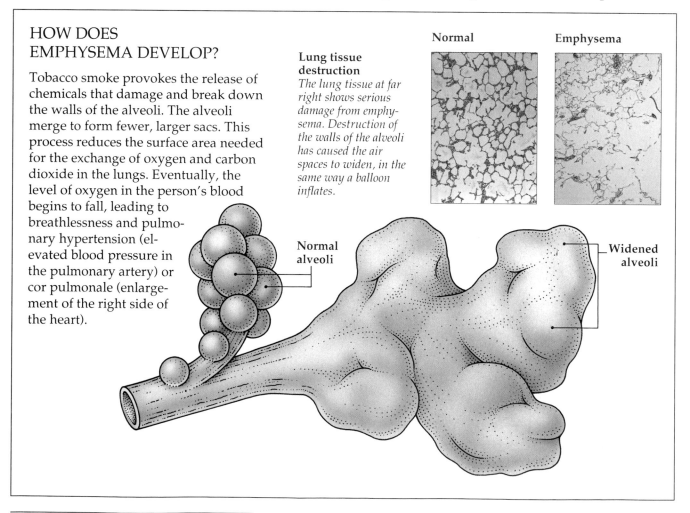

Normal

Emphysema

Normal alveoli

Widened alveoli

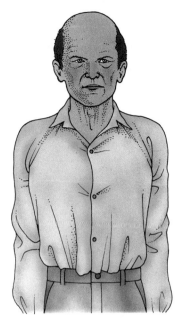

Thin and breathless
"Pink puffers" are usually thin and become breathless after slight activity. They breathe rapidly, exhale through pursed lips, and use their chest and neck muscles to help them breathe. They usually have an enlarged chest.

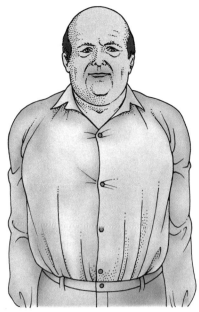

Overweight and bloated
"Blue bloaters" often have a severely low blood oxygen level that gives their lips and tongue a blue appearance. They tend to be overweight, may also be breathless, and have swollen ankles and abdomens from fluid retention.

Two profiles of people with emphysema

People with emphysema are sometimes described as "pink puffers" or "blue bloaters" because of their general appearance. "Pink puffers" usually do not seek medical care until they have experienced 5 to 10 years of progressive breathlessness, usually when they are about 60 years old or older. "Blue bloaters" tend to seek help at an earlier age, generally younger than 60, after many years of recurrent chest infections, coughing, phlegm production, and ankle swelling and other signs of congestive heart failure, including fluid retention and breathlessness.

Doctors do not know why people with chronic obstructive pulmonary disease fall into one of these categories. One theory suggests that the "blue and bloated" patients can tolerate the abnormal oxygen and carbon dioxide levels in their blood better than the "pink puffers," who must struggle for every breath. Many people show features of both types.

DIAGNOSING LUNG DISEASES

Doctors can usually diagnose emphysema and chronic bronchitis based on the findings of a physical examination, medical history, and lung function tests. These tests may also measure oxygen and carbon dioxide levels in the person's arterial blood.

ASK YOUR DOCTOR
BRONCHITIS AND EMPHYSEMA

Q My wife thinks that I should quit smoking because I have had a smokers' cough for years, which produces thick phlegm. Will quitting make a difference?

A Definitely. You probably have chronic bronchitis. If you continue smoking, you will develop irreversible and potentially crippling lung disease. If you quit, you will no longer cough and will stop further deterioration of your lungs.

Q My mother has severe emphysema. I have read that a nebulizer can sometimes help people with emphysema. What is a nebulizer, and do you think my mother would benefit from using one?

A Like an inhaler, a nebulizer delivers a drug in aerosol form, but it is easier to use. Inhaling bronchodilator drugs regularly through a nebulizer or an inhaler may improve breathing in some people with emphysema. Your mother should ask her doctor if a nebulizer would help her.

Q I have chronic obstructive pulmonary disease and am especially susceptible to chest infections in the winter. Aside from not smoking, is there anything I can do to prevent these chest infections?

A Keep your house and workplace warm and the humidity moderate. Stay indoors and avoid places where a lot of people gather. Your doctor may give you a reserve supply of antibiotics to take when you feel an infection coming on. But you must use the antibiotics only when necessary, because you could develop a resistance to them.

TREATMENT

People with chronic bronchitis or emphysema usually experience a steady decline in lung function and a worsening of symptoms, especially breathlessness. The rate of decline varies from person to person. No cure exists for chronic obstructive pulmonary disease, but certain measures can improve the quality and length of life of people who have it.

The first step you can take is to quit smoking. Consult your doctor immediately about respiratory tract infections, because these infections can be fatal in people with chronic obstructive pulmonary disease. The regular use of bronchodilator medication helps many people. Doctors also recommend a single vaccination against the pneumococcal bacteria and annual influenza vaccinations.

Medications

Bronchodilator drugs that relax bronchial smooth muscle and reduce inflammation may help people with chronic obstructive pulmonary disease. Corticosteroid drugs reduce breathlessness and wheezing in only a minority of people. Before recommending long-term corticosteroid treatment, a doctor will often prescribe them for a short time to find out if this treatment helps. Long-term use of corticosteroid drugs can have unwanted side effects, including demineralization (softening) of bones, stomach ulcers, and immune system suppression, which leaves the person more susceptible to infection.

Physical therapy

Relaxation techniques and breathing exercises may help reduce the sensation of breathlessness and improve the person's tolerance for exercise.

If mucous secretions are excessive, or if the person has difficulty clearing them, postural drainage techniques can help drain the accumulated secretions from the lungs (see page 121).

SUPPLEMENTAL OXYGEN

Breathing oxygen-enriched air at home can prolong the survival of people who have inadequate oxygen levels in their blood. But the person must use oxygen continuously for at least 15 hours each day to benefit. Oxygen for use at home can be stored as compressed gas in cylinders or as liquid oxygen in a tank. An oxygen concentrator (see below) can extract oxygen from the air. People can receive oxygen through small plastic tubes fastened near the opening of the nose. It can also be administered through a tube inserted into the trachea. People receiving oxygen must not smoke, not only because of the risk of fire, but also because it worsens their condition.

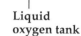

Liquid oxygen tank

Oxygen concentrator
Concentrators separate oxygen from the air. They are easy to install but require considerable electrical power to run. A concentrator eliminates the need for regular home deliveries of oxygen cylinders. A long, thin plastic tube (through which the oxygen flows) allows the person to move around.

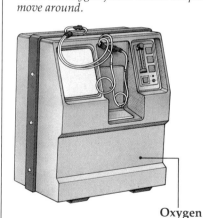

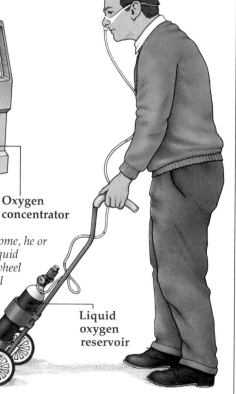

Oxygen concentrator

Portable oxygen
If the person wants to leave home, he or she can carry a reservoir of liquid oxygen over the shoulder or wheel it in a cart. The person can fill the reservoir from a large tank of oxygen at home (see above right). Pre-filled canisters containing smaller amounts of oxygen are also available for short-term use.

Liquid oxygen reservoir

CASE HISTORY
INCREASING BREATHLESSNESS

GERALD HAS BEEN a two-pack-a-day smoker since he was a teenager and has had a noticeable cough for the last 30 years. Recently, however, the cough became more persistent. Gerald also became concerned about increasing breathlessness that was preventing him from using stairs and even from walking quickly. He decided to talk to his doctor.

PERSONAL DETAILS
Name Gerald Hobbes
Age 63
Occupation Newspaper editor
Family Parents are dead.

MEDICAL BACKGROUND

Gerald started to cough, mainly during the winter, when he was a young man but he dismissed it as an inevitable "smokers' cough." Over the years, the cough has become more persistent. Recently, the cough has been almost as bad in the fall and spring as in the winter. Gerald has had many chest infections, especially in the winter, and his doctor has frequently prescribed antibiotics.

THE CONSULTATION

The doctor has been telling Gerald for years to stop smoking to avoid seriously damaging his lungs. The doctor is concerned but not surprised to hear about Gerald's worsening breathlessness and persistent cough.

THE DIAGNOSIS

From Gerald's symptoms and history, the doctor diagnoses CHRONIC OBSTRUCTIVE PULMONARY DISEASE. The doctor tells Gerald that this disease is a combination of chronic bronchitis and emphysema, resulting in a severe limitation of air flow. Cigarette smoke stimulates excess mucus production and causes persistent inflammation and narrowing of the airways (chronic bronchitis). Inhaled cigarette smoke also causes specialized white blood cells to release enzymes that digest and destroy the walls of the tiny air sacs in the lungs. This process impairs the efficiency with which oxygen can pass from the air in his lungs into his blood, a condition called emphysema.

THE DOCTOR'S ADVICE

The doctor tells Gerald that the most important thing he can do is to quit smoking immediately. If he stops right away, the chronic bronchitis with its cough and phlegm production will become less severe, and his breathlessness may also diminish.

THE FOLLOW-UP

Gerald does not stop smoking and his condition continues to deteriorate. After a few years, levels of oxygen in his blood fall so far that he needs to breathe oxygen from a tank. His doctor arranges for him to use an oxygen concentrator at home and prescribes a portable oxygen supply so he can leave his apartment and continue to receive oxygen. He has to retire from his job at the newspaper and becomes a semi-invalid.

THE OUTCOME

In spite of his disease, and against his doctor's warnings, Gerald continues to smoke. He even turns off his oxygen so that he can smoke. He becomes unable to leave his bed and dies of respiratory failure.

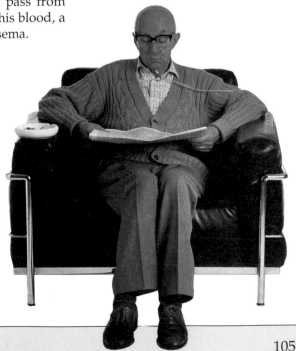

Breathing oxygen-enriched air
Gerald must breathe oxygen-enriched air for 15 hours every day, delivered by a catheter in the nose. Soft plastic prongs extend about 1/4 inch into each nostril. The prongs do not interfere with speech, eating, or drinking.

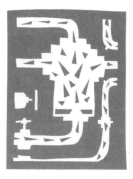

CIRCULATORY LUNG DISORDERS

MANY DISORDERS CAN AFFECT the circulation of blood to and from your lungs. Smoking damages both the circulatory system and the lungs. Doctors can treat circulatory or lung problems with drugs. But prevention of these disorders is much more effective. The best way to prevent such disorders is to refrain from smoking.

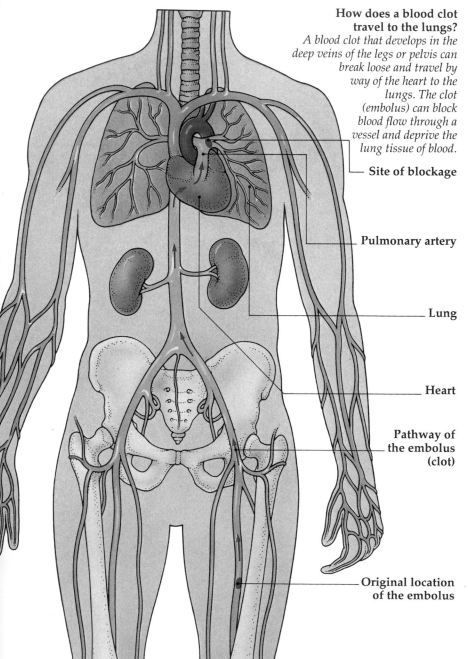

How does a blood clot travel to the lungs?
A blood clot that develops in the deep veins of the legs or pelvis can break loose and travel by way of the heart to the lungs. The clot (embolus) can block blood flow through a vessel and deprive the lung tissue of blood.

— Site of blockage

— Pulmonary artery

— Lung

— Heart

Pathway of the embolus (clot)

— Original location of the embolus

Your heart pumps blood to and from your lungs to replenish the blood with oxygen before sending it to the rest of your body. Any disruption in the passage of blood between your heart and lungs can seriously affect the level of oxygen in your blood. The circulation of blood through your lungs starts with the right side of your heart, where the blood is low in oxygen. Your heart pumps this oxygen-deficient blood through your pulmonary arteries into the capillaries of your lungs. The blood then picks up oxygen from the alveoli in your lungs and flows back to the left side of your heart by way of the pulmonary veins. From there, your heart pumps the blood out through the aorta to supply the rest of your body. Conditions affecting the pulmonary circulation can either develop suddenly or progress slowly over many years. Three of the most serious disorders are pulmonary embolism, pulmonary hypertension, and cor pulmonale.

PULMONARY EMBOLISM

A pulmonary embolism is a blockage of one or more divisions of the pulmonary artery. It usually occurs when a blood clot that has formed in a vein in the legs or pelvis breaks off and travels through the bloodstream to the lungs. When a clot travels from its site of origin, doctors call it an embolus. Clots in the legs may cause symptoms, such as swelling and pain, in the affected leg. But sometimes

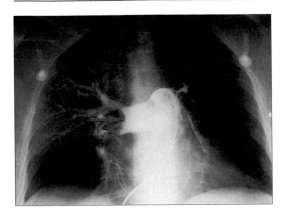

Embolus in the lungs
The pulmonary angiogram above shows a blood clot, called an embolus, causing a blockage in the right pulmonary artery (arrow).

clots cause no obvious symptoms.

Many factors can contribute to the formation of blood clots. The most dangerous factor is sluggish blood flow through the veins of the legs or pelvis. Sluggish blood flow occurs during immobility, such as prolonged bed rest, prolonged sitting (as during bus or plane trips), or a major surgical procedure. Other risk factors include injury to a vein in the pelvis or legs, burns to the lower limbs, pregnancy, obesity, cancer, heart failure, taking drugs that contain estrogen in high doses, being over the age of 70, and a few rare diseases in which the blood clots more easily than normal.

Warning signs
The most common symptom of pulmonary embolism is sudden breathlessness. Other symptoms include chest pain, palpitations, coughing up blood-stained phlegm, a slight fever, and wheezing. If you notice any of these symptoms, especially after surgery, bed rest, or prolonged immobility, consult your doctor.

Investigations
Blood test results and chest X-rays often appear normal in people who have pulmonary embolism, although the doctor may see signs of reduced blood flow through the affected lung. An electrocardiogram (a recording of the heart's electrical impulses) can sometimes help doctors distinguish pulmonary embolism from other causes of breathlessness and chest pain, such as asthma or a heart attack. Doctors usually perform V/Q lung scans (see page 77) to visualize the pattern of the blood and air flow through the lungs. If the V/Q scan does not rule out pulmonary embolism, then doctors may perform a pulmonary angiogram (shown at left) to confirm the diagnosis. The technique of angiography is described on page 77.

Treatment
When a doctor suspects pulmonary embolism, he or she begins drug treatment immediately, often before all test results are in. Treatment begins with the drug heparin, which keeps the person's blood from coagulating. Doctors prefer to administer the drug into the person's vein as a continuous infusion (drip), but they sometimes inject it under the skin every 4 to 6 hours. Heparin prevents further clotting but does not break down a clot that has already formed. Treatment with clot-dissolving drugs, such as streptokinase, helps people with large emboli. Doctors must occasionally remove blood clots surgically.

Once the person's condition stabilizes, doctors start treatment with an anticoagulant drug that can be taken by mouth, such as warfarin, after 5 to 7 days of heparin therapy. The oral drug replaces the heparin and clot-dissolving medications.

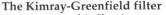

The Kimray-Greenfield filter
Doctors insert this filter into one of the venae cavae (the major veins in the body) to trap recurrent emboli from the legs or pelvis before they reach the lungs and cause damage. The device is just over an inch long.

DEEP VEIN THROMBOSIS
Doctors can perform several tests to confirm the presence of a blood clot (thrombus) in the deep veins of the legs or pelvis. Doctors can map the flow of blood through the veins with ultrasonic (high-frequency sound) energy and by measuring the electrical forces generated when the blood pushes against a clot. Neither test requires surgery. Both are simple and safe. To further confirm the presence of a blood clot in the veins, especially in the pelvic veins, doctors may perform venous angiography. During this procedure, doctors inject a contrast medium (see page 76) – through which X-rays cannot pass – into the veins of the person's foot. The pattern made when the veins fill with contrast medium is recorded on X-ray film.

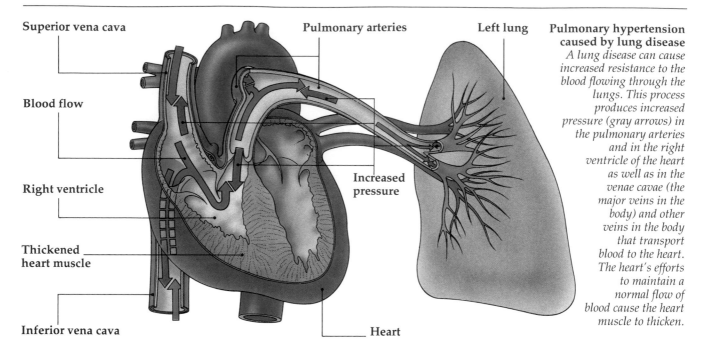

Superior vena cava

Blood flow

Right ventricle

Thickened heart muscle

Inferior vena cava

Pulmonary arteries

Left lung

Increased pressure

Heart

Pulmonary hypertension caused by lung disease
A lung disease can cause increased resistance to the blood flowing through the lungs. This process produces increased pressure (gray arrows) in the pulmonary arteries and in the right ventricle of the heart as well as in the venae cavae (the major veins in the body) and other veins in the body that transport blood to the heart. The heart's efforts to maintain a normal flow of blood cause the heart muscle to thicken.

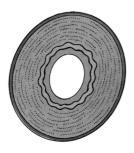

Early stages of pulmonary hypertension
The walls of the pulmonary artery are beginning to thicken.

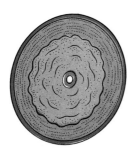

Later stages of pulmonary hypertension
The walls of the pulmonary artery are thickened with muscle and fibrous tissue.

PULMONARY HYPERTENSION

Pulmonary hypertension occurs when the blood pressure in the arteries leading to the lungs (pulmonary arteries) rises above a certain level. The hypertension may start on its own (primary hypertension) or be caused by an underlying condition (secondary hypertension).

Causes

The causes of primary pulmonary hypertension remain unknown. It is a rare disease that most commonly occurs in females between the ages of 10 and 40.

Secondary pulmonary hypertension is much more common and is produced by an underlying lung or heart disorder, or by a disease of the veins in the legs or arms. Lung diseases such as emphysema destroy lung tissue, impairing blood flow and increasing pressure in the pulmonary arteries. Heart failure, primarily in the chambers of the left side of the heart, leads to pulmonary hypertension. In people with heart failure, the heart cannot pump blood efficiently to the rest of the body, because of blockages in the arteries of the heart or because of diseased heart valves or heart muscle. A larger-than-normal volume of blood builds up in the lungs and causes increased blood pressure in the pulmonary arteries.

Warning signs

When a doctor examines a person for primary pulmonary hypertension, he or she detects few signs of disease. The doctor may hear abnormal heart sounds caused by the higher pressure that the heart must maintain to keep blood circulating through the person's lungs. In the later stages of the disease, the right side of the person's heart may fail (see COR PULMONALE on page 109).

The warning signs of secondary pulmonary hypertension depend on the underlying disease. For example, people with heart disease often experience breathlessness.

Tests and treatment

Doctors diagnose primary pulmonary hypertension by excluding all other possible causes of the disorder. Tests include a chest X-ray, which in later stages of the disease shows enlarged pulmonary arteries. An electrocardiogram may show evidence of the increased strain placed

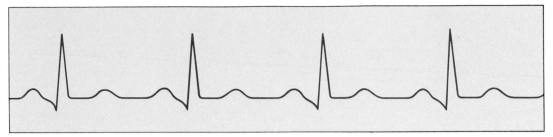

Normal ECG
This tracing is from a normally functioning heart. It shows the electrical impulses produced by healthy heart muscle.

on the right side of the heart. Doctors perform additional tests to exclude other lung diseases.

The treatment for primary pulmonary hypertension is not very effective. Drugs delivered through a catheter to the person's heart and major blood vessels widen the arteries and reduce the pressure in the pulmonary circulation. If drug treatment fails, doctors may consider a heart-lung transplant.

Treatment for secondary pulmonary hypertension focuses on controlling the underlying disease.

COR PULMONALE

Cor pulmonale is heart failure primarily of the right ventricle, caused by lung disease. This means that the chambers on the right side of the person's heart cannot pump enough blood to the lungs, causing blood to accumulate and pressure in the veins to rise.

Causes
The onset of cor pulmonale can be rapid when caused by a pulmonary embolus, respiratory failure from pneumonia, or asthma. In people with chronic pulmonary diseases such as chronic bronchitis, emphysema, and lung fibrosis (scarring), cor pulmonale develops gradually.

Warning signs
The first symptoms (usually breathlessness, coughing, and chest pain) are those of the underlying disease. Pressure from blood that has accumulated in the veins forces fluid out of the bloodstream into the tissues, causing enlargement of the liver and ankle swelling.

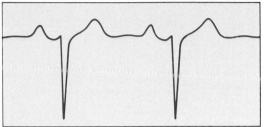

Abnormal ECG
This tracing shows a pattern typical of cor pulmonale. There is a reversal of the impulses shown above, suggesting enlargement of the right ventricle.

Tests and treatment
Doctors initially order tests, such as a chest X-ray and an electrocardiogram (ECG), to diagnose the underlying cause of the disease. Doctors then treat the underlying cause of the right-sided heart failure. Treatments include antibiotics for chronic bronchitis and pneumonia, bronchodilators for asthma, and anticoagulant drugs for pulmonary emboli. If blood oxygen levels are low, doctors order supplemental oxygen to lower the pressure in the pulmonary arteries, which reduces the work required from the heart. Doctors also prescribe diuretics, which are drugs that reduce the amount of fluid in the body, to reduce swelling.

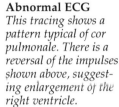

Effects of cor pulmonale
When the right side of the heart cannot efficiently pump blood, less blood leaves the heart (thin arrows) than enters it (thick blue arrows). This imbalance produces pressure in the veins (gray arrows). The liver and ankles swell from fluid collection.

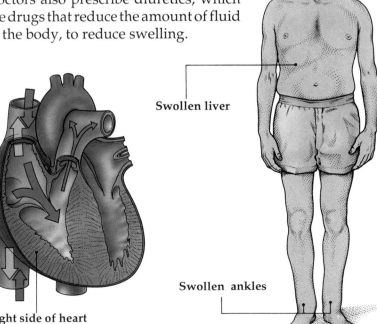

Swollen liver

Swollen ankles

**Right side of heart
(walls are abnormally thickened)**

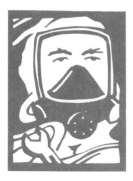

OCCUPATIONAL LUNG DISEASES

WHETHER YOU WORK in an office, in a factory, or on a farm, you may be exposed to occupational hazards that can affect your respiratory system. By knowing the sources of these hazards, wearing protective clothing, and taking precautions, you will be able to avoid serious damage to your respiratory system.

SILO-FILLERS' LUNG

Inhaling gases generated by feed stored in a silo can cause a condition called silo-fillers' lung. Symptoms include sudden fever, breathlessness, and wheezing caused by fluid in the lungs. This condition can be a medical emergency requiring hospitalization. Treatment includes oxygen, mechanical breathing assistance, and drugs.

The causes of some occupational lung problems are obvious, such as inhaling a toxic gas that produces difficulty breathing. But many lung diseases, such as silicosis (see page 112), common among foundry workers, and asbestosis, found in shipyard workers, can produce symptoms years after initial exposure to an irritant. This delay makes it more difficult for doctors to identify the cause.

GASES, FUMES, AND CHEMICALS

When people inhale gases, vapors, and fumes at work (see below), these substances can irritate or damage their airways or lungs. Inhaling toxic chemicals in the form of dust particles or powders can also cause lung damage. Examples of such chemicals include anhydrides (used in the chemical industry), zinc chloride powder and cobalt (used in the manufacture of metal alloys), and other metal salts, such as those containing mercury, cadmium, and nickel.

A person who realizes he or she has inhaled a potentially toxic substance should immediately seek medical care. Sometimes symptoms caused by inflammation of the bronchi, such as choking and breathlessness, develop immediately. Damage to the person's lungs can be permanent, resulting in breathlessness and wheezing. Severe lung injury can be fatal.

Where do irritant gases come from?
Gases that can irritate or damage a person's airways and lungs on the job include sulfur dioxide from oil refineries (below) and power plants, ammonia in fertilizers and explosives, and industrial gases such as chlorine, ozone, phosgene, and nitrogen dioxide.

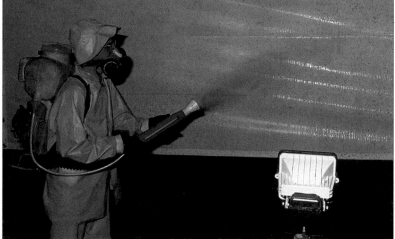

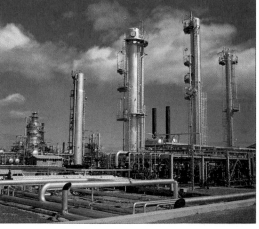

Protection against damaging fumes
Damaging fumes, such as those from insecticide sprays, can expose workers to respiratory tract damage. Canister-type masks and supplied-air breathing devices protect workers from such fumes, vapors, and aerosols.

EFFECTS OF GASES, FUMES, AND CHEMICALS

Gases, fumes, and chemicals can affect your respiratory system in the following ways:

Inflammation of nasal lining
The lining of your nose can become inflamed by chemicals such as chlorine and ammonia.

Spasm in the bronchi
Any irritant gas can cause a spasm in your bronchi that constricts your airways, producing wheezing and difficulty breathing.

Injury to cells lining the airways
Some inhaled gases can damage the cells that line your airways.

Inflammation and damage of air sacs
Inhaling noxious gases (such as ammonia) or metal salts (such as cobalt) can damage or inflame the lining of your alveoli (the small air sacs in your lungs).

Pulmonary edema
Lung damage caused by inhaling noxious gases or chemicals can cause pulmonary edema (fluid accumulation in your lungs), leading to difficulty breathing.

Fibrosis
Lung damage with fibrosis (scar tissue formation) can occur after inhalation of toxic chemicals or materials.

Bleeding in the lungs
Inhaling high doses of certain chemicals can cause bleeding in your lungs.

Entry into the bloodstream
Molecules from inhaled fumes can enter the bloodstream, causing widespread damage in the body.

Lung cell damage from paraquat
Inhaling the weed killer paraquat can cause lung cells to burst, producing inflammation and, eventually, scarring.

SMOKE INHALATION

Firefighters and other people in or near a fire risk lung and airway damage from smoke inhalation. Burning wood produces very acidic smoke, which can injure the lungs. Often, the most severe damage comes from inhaling chemicals released from burning materials (see right). Water used to put out the fire can produce suspended water droplets that contain chemicals from the burning materials. When inhaled, these droplets can cause severe lung damage.

A person who has been overcome by smoke must be removed from the vicinity of the fire. Even if a person seems unaffected immediately after exposure to smoke, respiratory problems could develop during the next 24 hours.

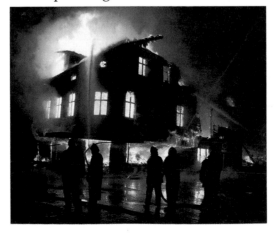

Danger from burning materials
During a fire, burning wood, paper, cotton, and plastic release harmful chemicals. If a person inhales smoke containing these chemicals, severe lung damage can result.

PNEUMOCONIOSES

Pneumoconiosis literally means "dust lung." The lung diseases known as pneumoconioses are caused by inhaling irritating mineral or metal particles, such as those of silica, coal, asbestos, beryllium, or cobalt. These inhaled particles irritate and inflame lung tissue, producing lung damage and fibrosis (formation of scar tissue). Once fibrosis has occurred, the diseases are irreversible.

Silicosis

Lung fibrosis induced by inhaling silica dust, usually in the form of quartz, is called silicosis. This disorder is the most common occupational disease in the world. Exposure to the dust may have been brief but intense. It can be many years before symptoms develop.

The main symptom of silicosis is breathlessness, sometimes accompanied by a cough. Small, rounded shadows seen on a chest X-ray indicate the start of fibrosis. At this stage, the person may not yet have symptoms. Later, lung function becomes severely restricted. Silicosis can lead to lung cancer, especially if the person with silicosis smokes.

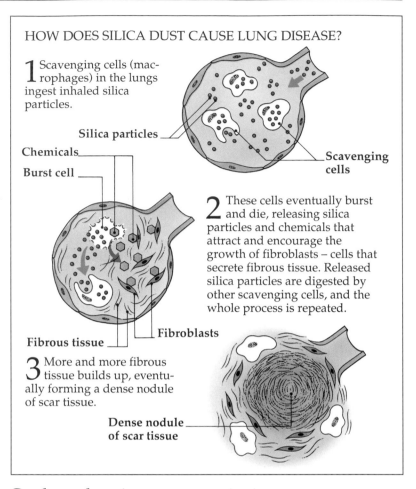

HOW DOES SILICA DUST CAUSE LUNG DISEASE?

1 Scavenging cells (macrophages) in the lungs ingest inhaled silica particles.

Silica particles

Chemicals

Burst cell

Scavenging cells

2 These cells eventually burst and die, releasing silica particles and chemicals that attract and encourage the growth of fibroblasts – cells that secrete fibrous tissue. Released silica particles are digested by other scavenging cells, and the whole process is repeated.

Fibrous tissue

Fibroblasts

3 More and more fibrous tissue builds up, eventually forming a dense nodule of scar tissue.

Dense nodule of scar tissue

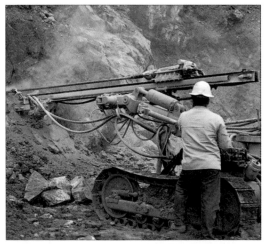

Danger from a widely used mineral
Silica, which causes the disease called silicosis, is commonly found in sand and rock. People at risk of silicosis include quarry workers (above), mine workers, sand blasters, ceramic workers, stone masons, grinders, and polishers.

Coal workers' pneumoconiosis

A coal miner may have both coal workers' pneumoconiosis, also known as "black lung disease," and silicosis if the coal being mined is rich in quartz. Coal dust, inhaled regularly during a period of at least 10 to 15 years, becomes deposited in lung tissue and causes the lungs to form nodules. Scar tissue (fibrosis) forms around the nodules, causing further destruction of the surrounding lung tissue. In people with silicosis and coal workers' pneumoconiosis, a large mass of scar tissue called progressive massive fibrosis can form if many nodules merge.

Symptoms are often absent early in the course of coal workers' pneumoconiosis – except for chronic bronchitis induced by the dust, often greatly exaggerated by smoking. Later, when scarring has interfered with the flow of blood to the lungs, breathlessness and damage to the right side of the heart can develop.

Pneumoconiosis
The specimen of lung tissue below was taken from a person who had pneumoconiosis. The numerous black spots are particles of coal dust. In pneumoconiosis, areas of fibrosis (scar tissue) build up around these particles.

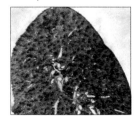

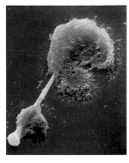

Unsuccessful defense
In the lungs, scavenging white blood cells called macrophages ingest inhaled asbestos fibers. The fibers destroy the cells, which release enzymes that cause inflammation and, eventually, fibrosis (scarring). The photograph above (magnified 1,300 times) shows two macrophages impaled on an asbestos fiber.

Asbestosis

Inhaling asbestos fibers causes scarring of the lung tissue. Doctors call this condition asbestosis. People at risk include those who are directly exposed to asbestos – such as shipyard, construction, and demolition workers, asbestos miners, and insulators – and people who are indirectly exposed to asbestos, such as electricians and plumbers. The major symptom of asbestosis is breathlessness.

Berylliosis

Berylliosis is a rare disease caused by exposure to the metal beryllium, which is used in the fluorescent light industry, in nuclear reactors, and in the space program. The effects of acute berylliosis include fibrosis of lung tissue and pulmonary edema (see page 120). Symptoms of chronic berylliosis are breathlessness, coughing, chest pain, and joint pain. Doctors think that inflammation and scarring are caused by a reaction of white blood cells to beryllium.

ALLERGIC REACTIONS TO ORGANIC SUBSTANCES

Allergic reactions to organic substances may follow inhalation of dusts from unprocessed cotton (byssinosis), sugar cane (bagassosis), and flour (bakers' asthma). Similar conditions are bird handlers' disease and maple bark disease. Such reactions may be caused by bacterial contamination of the inhaled products. Lung function can become permanently impaired. Symptoms, including breathlessness and chest tightness, usually improve when the person avoids exposure to the dusts. Inhaling bronchodilator drugs and improved working conditions, including dust extraction, may help the person relieve symptoms.

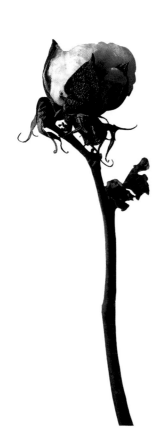

Hazard for cotton workers
The lung disease byssinosis has been prevalent for at least 250 years. Doctors believe inhaling dusts from unprocessed cotton causes the disease.

ASK YOUR DOCTOR
OCCUPATIONAL LUNG DISEASES

Q I have worked as a pipe fitter for 5 years. My job exposes me to the asbestos in pipe insulation. How can I avoid getting asbestosis in the future?

A Current occupational safety and health regulations protect workers from exposure to hazardous substances such as asbestos if workers follow the rules. You should always wear a protective suit and gloves and a canister-type face mask while working so that you will not inhale any asbestos fibers from the air and to prevent the fibers from settling on your skin and clothing.

Q My son and I are farmers. We have been having repeated attacks of fever, chills, and coughing after it rains. Could these symptoms be related to our farm work?

A Exposure to moldy hay that contains a growing fungus sometimes produces the symptoms you describe. Doctors call this disorder farmers' lung. Symptoms usually start 4 to 8 hours after exposure to the fungus, which grows more rapidly after a heavy rain.

Q I have asthma and it seems to be getting worse. Could my job cleaning houses be making my asthma worse?

A Possibly. If your asthma gets worse while you are working and improves when you are not, it is probably being aggravated by exposure to something you come into contact with at work, such as dust. Your doctor can perform tests to find out which allergens present at your job are triggering your asthma.

OCCUPATIONAL ASTHMA

More than 100 chemicals in the workplace can cause asthma (see right). In addition, people who already have asthma may find that their symptoms become worse when they are exposed to certain materials at work.

The reasons some people develop asthma when exposed to these agents remain unclear, but doctors think an exaggerated immune or allergic response might be involved. The affected person usually has symptoms typical of asthma, such as wheezing, chest tightness, and a cough, which generally improve when they do not work.

Doctors usually advise the person to avoid or minimize exposure to the chemical and prescribe bronchodilator drugs (see page 96) that the person can inhale to relieve narrowing of the airways.

HYPERSENSITIVITY PNEUMONITIS

Hypersensitivity pneumonitis is lung inflammation that develops in a person who has an unusually high sensitivity to an inhaled substance. The disease probably arises from an immune or allergic reaction to the substance, not from infection by an organism.

Occupational asthma culprits
Substances that can cause occupational asthma include toluene (found in paints and polyurethane foam), grain dust, wood dust from the Western red cedar, industrial chemicals such as trimetallic anhydrides and platinum salts, and dusts from various animals and plants.

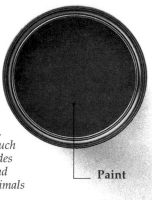

Paint

Wood dust

The person usually develops a fever, a cough, chills, and breathlessness about 4 to 6 hours after inhaling the offending material. Repeated exposure can cause weight loss, weakness, emphysema (see page 102), or lung fibrosis (scarring).

Many substances can cause hypersensitivity pneumonitis. Doctors have given the disease different names, some based on occupations that have exposed people to agents that have caused the disease. Examples of these names include farmers' lung, caused by fungal spores released from moldy hay, and malt workers' lung, caused by fungal contaminants contained in barley. Some chemicals can also cause hypersensitivity pneumonitis.

After the diagnosis, the doctor advises the affected person to avoid or reduce exposure to the agent. A protective face mask can help reduce exposure to some agents but is not completely effective. Sometimes affected people must change jobs to avoid further exposure. Treatment with corticosteroid drugs may relieve severe symptoms. Some people need treatment with oxygen.

Hazards of bird handling
Pigeon-breeders' lung and turkey handlers' disease are types of occupational asthma. In some people, inhaling proteins found in the birds' droppings or feathers causes hypersensitivity pneumonitis.

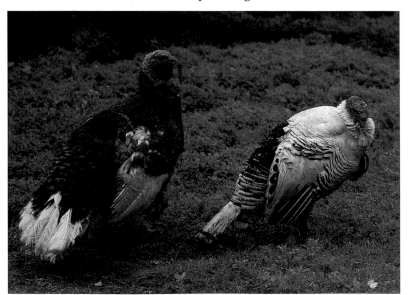

CASE HISTORY
DIFFICULTY BREATHING

RECENTLY, WAYNE BECAME **aware of having to stop to catch his breath after climbing each flight of stairs in his apartment building. He initially attributed this breathlessness to smoking a pack of cigarettes a day and decided to cut down. But even after cutting down, he began to have great difficulty breathing when he walked. Wayne decided to see his doctor.**

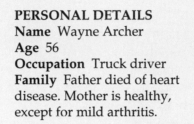

PERSONAL DETAILS
Name Wayne Archer
Age 56
Occupation Truck driver
Family Father died of heart disease. Mother is healthy, except for mild arthritis.

MEDICAL BACKGROUND
Wayne has smoked for many years, but he has been healthy until recently. He does not enjoy exercise and pays little attention to his diet, so he considers himself lucky to have been healthy for so long.

Taking the chest X-ray
Wayne stands with his hands behind his back. The X-ray technician positions his chest next to a screen that contains photographic film. The X-ray beams pass through Wayne's chest and lungs to create an image on the film.

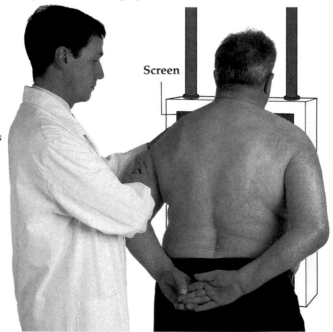

Screen

THE CONSULTATION
The doctor questions Wayne about his symptoms and asks where he has worked. Wayne tells the doctor that he worked in a coal mine between the ages of 17 and 38. During the physical examination, the doctor finds that the right side of Wayne's heart is not working properly. He suspects that Wayne might have a heart condition called cor pulmonale that can be caused by an underlying lung disease.

FURTHER INVESTIGATION
The doctor orders a chest X-ray. The results show an enlarged heart and extensive lung fibrosis (scar tissue), which is restricting the entry of oxygen into Wayne's bloodstream. The doctor refers Wayne to a chest specialist, who performs tests that measure how much air is passing into and out of Wayne's lungs and the rate at which his bloodstream absorbs an inhaled gas. The results confirm that Wayne's symptoms are caused by lung disease.

THE DIAGNOSIS
Although it has been many years since Wayne worked in the coal mine, coal dust deposits remaining in his lungs have probably caused the lung fibrosis. Doctors call this condition COAL WORKERS' PNEUMOCONIOSIS, or black lung disease. Wayne's history of smoking has undoubtedly worsened his symptoms.

THE TREATMENT
Although no treatment can reverse Wayne's lung fibrosis, some steps can help the chronic bronchitis that developed from his cigarette smoking. Wayne quits smoking, because continued smoking will worsen his condition. The doctor prescribes an inhaled bronchodilator drug to help widen Wayne's airways and tells Wayne to use it whenever he becomes breathless.

THE OUTCOME
Wayne's condition does not improve very much, and he has to retire early from his job.

LUNG TISSUE DISORDERS

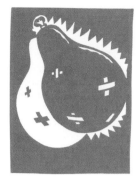

YOUR AIRWAYS AND THE BLOOD VESSELS in your lungs are surrounded and supported by tissue called the interstitium. Conditions, such as scarring, that affect this tissue are called interstitial lung diseases. Some disorders, such as cystic fibrosis and sarcoidosis, affect not only lung tissue but also many other parts of the body, including the liver, spleen, pancreas, and nervous system.

Recent advances by cellular and molecular biologists have contributed to our understanding of the ways in which lung tissue disorders develop.

of known cause, such as environmental lung diseases (see OCCUPATIONAL LUNG DISEASES on page 110), and those of unknown cause. When interstitial lung disease of unknown cause is accompanied by scarring, doctors call the condition idiopathic pulmonary fibrosis.

INTERSTITIAL LUNG DISEASES

Diseases that affect the deep lung tissue (interstitium) are chronic and slowly progressive disorders that the affected person may be unaware of for many years. When the lungs become distorted and scarred with fibrous tissue, the person becomes short of breath and eventually cannot get enough oxygen.

Because almost 200 different conditions can affect the interstitium, interstitial lung diseases are difficult to classify. Sometimes doctors divide them into those

Idiopathic pulmonary fibrosis

People with idiopathic pulmonary fibrosis often have only mild symptoms, such as a dry cough and some shortness of breath, when first seen by a doctor. As the disease progresses and scarring of the lungs develops, the person becomes increasingly short of breath and fatigued. About half of all people with idiopathic pulmonary fibrosis lose weight because the lack of oxygen causes their bodies to burn more calories.

WHO GETS INTERSTITIAL LUNG DISEASES?

The average age of people with an interstitial lung disease is 50, although affected people can range from infants to older people. The diseases seem to run in families, leading researchers to theorize that a genetic factor may be the cause in some people.

HOW DOES IDIOPATHIC PULMONARY FIBROSIS DEVELOP?

Doctors believe that inflammation, caused by substances released from the breakdown of normal white blood cells, plays a role in the development of this disease.

1 In the early stages of idiopathic pulmonary fibrosis, an increase in the number of white blood cells occurs in the lungs. The white blood cells secrete substances that cause constant inflammation.

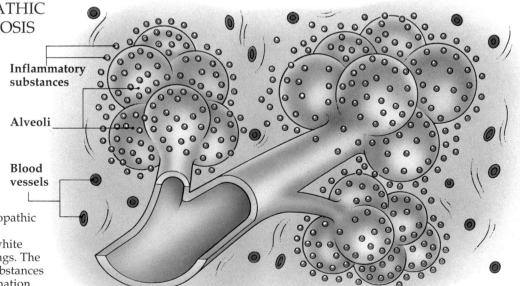

Inflammatory substances

Alveoli

Blood vessels

HOW DO DOCTORS DIAGNOSE IDIOPATHIC PULMONARY FIBROSIS?

After taking the person's medical history and performing a physical examination, the doctor will order a chest X-ray and perform pulmonary function tests (see page 78). Accurate diagnosis often requires the examination of a piece of lung tissue under a microscope. Doctors usually obtain the specimen with a fiberoptic bronchoscope (see page 80). An analysis of lung cells (see right) may help determine the degree of inflammation. If the diagnosis remains in doubt, doctors may perform an operation to obtain a sample of lung tissue for examination and analysis.

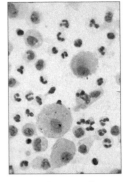

Normal   **Abnormal**

Analyzing lung cells
Normal tissue (above left) contains mainly one type of white blood cell, scavenger cells called macrophages. Inflamed tissue has fewer, but larger macrophages (the three large cells in the photograph above right). Both photographs are magnified 100 times.

OTHER TYPES OF INTERSTITIAL LUNG DISEASES

Some interstitial lung diseases seem to be related to collagen vascular diseases, a group of disorders of unknown cause that affect the whole body. Collagen is a tough, fibrous protein – the most common protein in your body. Collagen vascular diseases include rheumatoid arthritis and systemic lupus erythematosus. These diseases are characterized by immune system malfunctioning that affects blood vessels. The scarring produced by certain collagen vascular diseases accompanies bleeding in the lungs and kidney disease. Affected people may cough up blood, become anemic, and have poor kidney function.

Treatment

The treatment of idiopathic pulmonary fibrosis depends on the severity of the disease and the individual response to medication, but all affected people must first stop smoking. In some people, corticosteroid drugs (such as prednisone) or drugs that suppress the immune system help decrease lung inflammation and halt progression of the disease. For a person with very severe lung tissue scarring, oxygen may alleviate shortness of breath. Lung damage can cause heart failure, which leads to further breathing problems. Treatment with specific drugs is sometimes effective. People with progressive disease that does not respond to drugs or other therapy and who are otherwise in good health may be considered for lung transplantation surgery (see page 123). Most people with idiopathic pulmonary fibrosis die when their lungs become filled with scar tissue, or from heart failure.

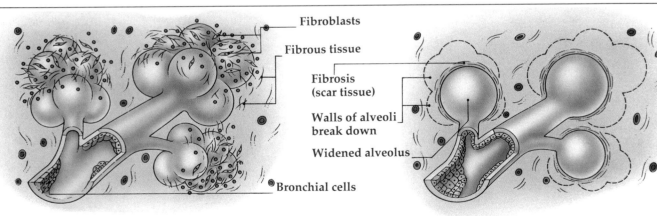

2 The substances secreted by the white blood cells activate cells called fibroblasts, which cause growth of the fibrous tissue of the lung. Overgrowth of fibrous tissue leads to lung scarring (fibrosis) that interferes with the exchange of oxygen and carbon dioxide. Overgrowth of bronchial cells also limits air flow.

3 Scar tissue eventually surrounds the alveoli, the walls of some alveoli break down, and the remaining alveoli widen. Considerable distortion of the lung can occur when the scar tissue contracts. Scar tissue can also restrict the expansion and contraction of the lung.

SARCOIDOSIS

Sarcoidosis is a disease of unknown cause that affects many organs throughout the body in addition to the lungs. Most doctors believe that sarcoidosis is caused by a heightened immune response to a foreign substance or to one of the body's own proteins. In the US, the prevalence of sarcoidosis ranges from 10 to 40 per 100,000 of the population. For reasons that are not understood, most affected people are black.

Diagnosis and treatment

Doctors base diagnosis of sarcoidosis on findings of a physical examination and the results of diagnostic tests, including a chest X-ray and lung biopsy (removal and examination of lung tissue). No blood test exists to diagnose sarcoidosis, but certain tests may help determine how the person will respond to treatment. In about half of all cases, the disease goes away by itself without any treatment. In some cases, the doctor prescribes corticosteroid drugs, such as prednisone, which suppress the body's abnormal immune activity. If sarcoidosis is mainly limited to the lungs, doctors will observe the patient for several months and review the results of a series of chest X-rays and lung function tests to see whether the person's condition is improving or getting worse.

Most people who have the sudden, short-term form of the disease recover fully. In 15 to 20 percent of people, the disease remains active or recurs. Sarcoidosis is fatal in 10 percent of cases.

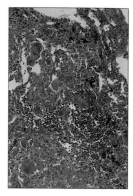

Granulomas
Sarcoidosis is characterized by accumulations of cells, called granulomas (shown here magnified 74 times), that may be interspersed with fibrous material in the body. Granulomas serve as a defense against allergens, irritants, or microorganisms.

HOW DOES SARCOIDOSIS AFFECT THE BODY?

Sarcoidosis can affect all parts of the body, but it affects the lungs and lymph glands in 90 percent of all people with the disease. In about a fourth of those with sarcoidosis, the disease affects the skin and eyes. Other systems are less commonly affected. People most often experience mild early symptoms affecting the lungs, but in some people, the disease develops rapidly, and generalized symptoms of fatigue, loss of appetite, and fever accompany respiratory symptoms. Other people develop respiratory symptoms very gradually and usually do not experience fever and fatigue.

Nervous system
Sarcoidosis can affect all parts of the nervous system. Temporary facial paralysis is a common symptom.

Joints
Arthritislike joint pain and swelling occur.

Lymph nodes
Most affected people have enlarged lymph nodes.

Liver
Although liver biopsies frequently reveal liver abnormalities, many affected people have few specific symptoms.

Bone marrow
Mild abnormalities of the blood can appear.

Eyes
Eye symptoms include blurred vision, watery eyes, and sensitivity to light.

Lungs
Respiratory symptoms can include coughing, shortness of breath, and a sensation of chest discomfort.

Skin
Skin inflammation and the appearance of red, raised nodules or abnormal patches can occur.

Spleen
The spleen may become enlarged.

CASE HISTORY
BREATHLESSNESS AT REST

DAN WAS ALWAYS **healthy and energetic. He played football in college and enjoyed skiing. But, at 27, he began to feel less and less physically fit. He became breathless even when he was not exerting himself and developed a persistent, dry cough. Gradually, he had to give up all sports. When it became difficult to get through a work day, Dan finally went to see his doctor.**

PERSONAL DETAILS
Name Dan Laughlin
Age 29
Occupation Computer service technician
Family Both parents are healthy. Dan has no personal history of respiratory disease.

MEDICAL BACKGROUND
Until he entered his late 20s, Dan enjoyed excellent health.

THE INITIAL CONSULTATION
Dan tells the doctor that he sometimes becomes breathless even when at rest and that he has been coughing for months. When he examines Dan, the doctor finds that his chest expands very little when he inhales and that his rate of breathing is unusually rapid. When he listens to Dan's breathing with his stethoscope, the doctor hears widespread, loud, crackling sounds in his chest toward the end of each inhalation. The doctor refers Dan to a chest specialist.

THE SPECIALIST'S CONSULTATION
The specialist questions Dan extensively about where he previously worked. Dan says that he has never been exposed to asbestos or other dusts. The doctor examines Dan and orders a chest X-ray.

FURTHER INVESTIGATION
Tests measuring how well Dan's lungs function show that there is good air flow into and out of Dan's lungs, but that his lungs cannot hold much air. The amount of oxygen in his blood is below normal and drops even further during mild exertion. The doctor uses a bronchoscope to obtain samples of Dan's lung tissue and fluid from his bronchus and sends them to the laboratory for examination under a microscope.

THE DIAGNOSIS AND TREATMENT
The results of the X-ray and the abnormal appearance of the lung tissue and fluid samples confirm that Dan has IDIOPATHIC PULMONARY FIBROSIS. This disease, of unknown cause, produces fibrous scar tissue (fibrosis) in the lungs, making the passage of oxygen into the blood increasingly difficult. When the scar tissue contracts, the lungs become stiff and cannot expand or contract.

The doctor initially treats Dan with corticosteroid drugs, which are effective in about one third of all people with the disease. After 6 weeks, Dan's condition has not improved, and he begins to show side effects (such as acne, swollen ankles, and elevated blood pressure) from the corticosteroid drugs. The doctor gradually discontinues the drug therapy.

THE FOLLOW-UP
Dan soon needs continuous oxygen therapy. Within weeks, signs of increasing resistance to the blood flow through his lungs begin to appear, and the doctors fear that the right side of Dan's heart might fail. The doctors decide to perform a double lung transplant while Dan's heart remains healthy. Fortunately, they are able to find a suitable donor.

THE OUTCOME
After Dan's operation, several complications arise, including infection. But, within a few days, his condition improves. He continues to get stronger and, by the next winter, Dan returns to work.

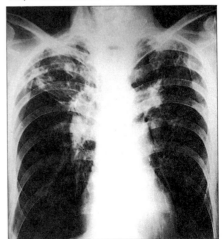

Chest X-ray
Dan's lungs look more opaque than healthy lungs, especially in the upper portions, as shown on the X-ray above. The dense white streaks represent areas of scar tissue that parallel the airways.

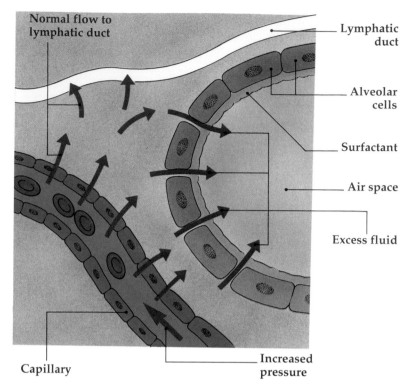

Normal flow to lymphatic duct

Lymphatic duct

Alveolar cells

Surfactant

Air space

Excess fluid

Capillary

Increased pressure

Why does pulmonary edema happen?
In a healthy person, about 4 teaspoons of fluid flow from the lung's capillaries into the lung tissue every hour. The fluid drains into the person's lymphatic system and eventually returns to the blood vessels. If an increase in pressure inside the blood vessels occurs or if the capillaries become more porous, more fluid flows into the lung tissue, as shown above. Excess fluid may reach the air spaces in the alveoli if the pressure is high enough to force fluid between the cells of the alveoli and through the layer of surfactant (see page 28) that lines them.

PULMONARY EDEMA

Pulmonary edema refers to the presence of excess fluid in the lungs, regardless of the cause. Causes of pulmonary edema can include increased pressure or leaking of fluid from the capillaries (tiny blood vessels) of the lungs (see above). The most common cause of pulmonary edema from increased capillary pressure is heart failure, usually caused by heart disease, diseases of the heart valves, or hypertension (high blood pressure). Increased capillary pressure can also be caused by other conditions, such as excess fluid in the bloodstream from kidney disease. Capillary leakage can result from inhaling either corrosive gases or vomit or may accompany severe pneumonia or shock.

A person who has pulmonary edema is short of breath and coughs up frothy, sometimes blood-streaked phlegm. Doctors can see pulmonary edema on a chest X-ray, but determining the cause can be difficult, particularly in older people who may have several medical conditions that could cause edema. Doctors treat pulmonary edema by trying to reverse the underlying cause. Other treatments include diuretics (drugs that encourage passage of fluid from the body) and oxygen therapy.

CYSTIC FIBROSIS

Cystic fibrosis is a genetic disorder that affects many organs in the body, especially the lungs and pancreas. The disorder appears only if a person has inherited two defective genes – one from each parent. The parents themselves are usually not affected by the disorder because they carry only one of the defective genes. In the US, about one child in every 2,000 is born with cystic fibrosis. The disorder causes the production of abnormal mucus throughout the body.

Symptoms

Cystic fibrosis causes mucus-secreting cells throughout the body to produce abnormally thick and sticky secretions. In the person's lungs, the thick mucus plugs up small airways, setting the stage for chronic infection and inflammation. Usually, the cilia (fine hairs that line the airways) sweep mucus secretions back up the airways to the trachea and carry away any bacteria or debris in the lungs. But, in people with cystic fibrosis, the secretions are so thick that the cilia cannot move them. The lung's normal defense mechanisms cannot clear away bacteria, and infections develop easily. The mucus-secreting cells respond to these infections by increasing their output, making it even harder for the person's body to dispose of the mucus. Eventually, after repeated infections, the lungs become damaged and scarred.

Other organs also secrete mucus, especially in the digestive system, which can cause problems for people with cystic fibrosis. For example, mucus can plug the pancreatic duct, preventing the normal secretion of digestive enzymes. This

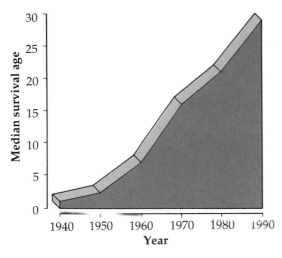

Survival of people with cystic fibrosis
Life expectancy for people with cystic fibrosis has soared, thanks to improved medical care. Many affected people now survive well into adulthood.

process hinders the absorption of nutrients from food and causes large, foul-smelling stools, and numerous bowel problems. The gallbladder and liver may also function improperly. Cystic fibrosis can affect the reproductive system, causing sterility in men.

Diagnosis

Doctors may not be able to diagnose some people who have only a mild case of cystic fibrosis until they reach adulthood. But the disease can sometimes be recognized in infancy. In newborns, the first sign may be blockage of the intestine, while in young children the first indications can be diarrhea, lack of expected growth, or a chest infection and a cough. In older children, symptoms usually include coughing, wheezing, weight loss, and diarrhea. Doctors confirm the diagnosis by measuring the salt content of the person's sweat. High levels of salt indicate cystic fibrosis.

Care and treatment

People with cystic fibrosis must clear the thick secretions from their airways through effective coughing. Percussion (clapping) of the person's chest with the hands loosens phlegm, and postural drainage (see right) helps bring it up.

Good nutrition is important, and bronchodilator drugs (which widen airways) may help some people. Controlling infections is critical for the person's long-term survival. People who develop infections often need antibiotics. Doctors perform double lung or heart-lung transplants for only a very few people with cystic fibrosis.

Loosening secretions
Percussion (clapping) of the chest or back with a cupped hand by another person may help loosen mucus in the affected person's lungs. Mechanical percussion devices are also available. "Huffing," breathing out forcibly while flapping the elbows, is another method of loosening mucus.

FUTURE TREATMENT

The genetic defect that causes cystic fibrosis has been identified recently. Scientists may soon develop drugs or a replacement for a substance in the body that people with cystic fibrosis lack to prevent the thick, sticky secretions that are characteristic of the disease. Gene replacement therapy could even lead to a permanent "cure."

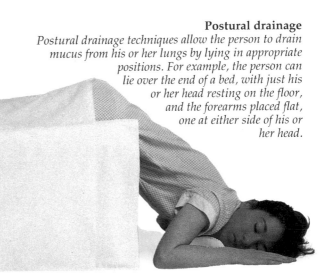

Postural drainage
Postural drainage techniques allow the person to drain mucus from his or her lungs by lying in appropriate positions. For example, the person can lie over the end of a bed, with just his or her head resting on the floor, and the forearms placed flat, one at either side of his or her head.

CASE HISTORY
AN UNDERWEIGHT BABY

For the first few months of her life, Sarah seemed to be a very healthy baby. But, by the time she was 8 months old, her mother, Louise, had became concerned about Sarah's health. Although the baby had a good appetite, she was not gaining weight and had begun to pass extremely pale, strong-smelling stools. Louise wondered whether Sarah might be suffering from a food allergy and took her to the doctor.

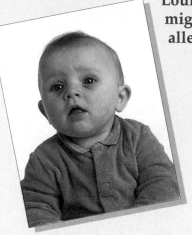

PERSONAL DETAILS
Name Sarah Arnott
Age 8 months
Family Sarah has a healthy 3-year-old brother. Her parents have no history of serious illness.

MEDICAL BACKGROUND
Sarah was born at full term after a vaginal delivery and was initially healthy. During the past 2 months, she has been treated for recurrent chest infections.

THE CONSULTATION
Louise explains to the doctor that Sarah is failing to gain weight and that her stools seem abnormal. She also mentions that Sarah seems to be getting more chest infections.

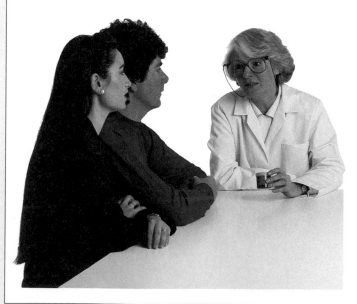

Diet advice
A nutritionist explains to Sarah's parents that their baby requires a diet high in calories and protein to help her gain weight. She shows them how to supplement Sarah's diet with capsules containing the digestive enzymes she lacks so that she can adequately digest and absorb her food.

The doctor finds that Sarah is indeed underweight and has a slightly distended stomach. When he listens to her chest through a stethoscope, the doctor hears chest congestion. He arranges for Sarah to have tests.

THE DIAGNOSIS
A blood test and a test that measures the salt content of Sarah's perspiration confirm that she has CYSTIC FIBROSIS, an inherited condition caused by a faulty gene. The disease causes abnormal amounts of salt in sweat and produces excessively sticky secretions that increase susceptibility to chest infections. It can also inhibit the secretion by the pancreas of enzymes necessary for adequate digestion, causing abnormal stools.

The doctor tells Sarah's parents that while Sarah possesses two copies of the defective gene that causes cystic fibrosis, they each have only one and are unaffected. He advises them to have genetic counseling before trying to conceive again.

THE TREATMENT
Sarah is only moderately affected by the disease, so the doctor thinks that she should be able to have a reasonably good quality of life, with treatment. The first goal of treatment is to make sure that Sarah receives adequate nutrition. The second goal is to prevent recurrent chest infections, using postural drainage to keep her chest free of sticky secretions. Prompt antibiotic treatment will be vital to minimize lung damage if she does develop an infection.

THE OUTLOOK
Sarah's parents help her gain weight and try their best to control her chest infections. But they realize that she may not survive past early adulthood unless new treatments become available.

LUNG TRANSPLANTATION

Doctors may consider lung transplantation for some people with irreversible lung disorders. Lung transplantation is available at only a few major medical centers in the US. Surgeons are still studying and refining the procedure. Donor organs are in very short supply.

When the procedure was first developed, a combined heart-lung transplant was the only way surgeons could successfully transplant lung tissue. Then surgeons developed a way to join the transplanted lung tissue to the recipient's vessels and trachea or bronchus without replacing his or her own healthy heart.

Suitable candidates for lung transplantation are people who have severe lung diseases, such as emphysema, which are progressive and no longer respond to conventional treatment. Candidates must not have any other diseases and must be prepared to undergo a physically and emotionally traumatic experience. Most lung transplant centers do not accept people who are older than 60.

People who have had a lung transplant, and who receive good follow-up care, have a good chance of surviving for up to 2 years. Long-term survival rates are not yet known.

SINGLE OR DOUBLE LUNG TRANSPLANTS?

Surgeons currently perform double lung transplants primarily for people who have cystic fibrosis. Single lung transplants are performed for people who have more common conditions, such as emphysema. Single lung transplants also make the most efficient use of scarce donor lungs.

Postoperative care
After surgery, the patient's breathing is maintained with a ventilator connected to an air tube inserted into the trachea. Drainage tubes inserted in the chest drain blood and fluid from the lungs. Drugs that suppress the immune system are given to prevent the recipient's body from rejecting the donated organs. These drugs increase susceptibility to lethal infections.

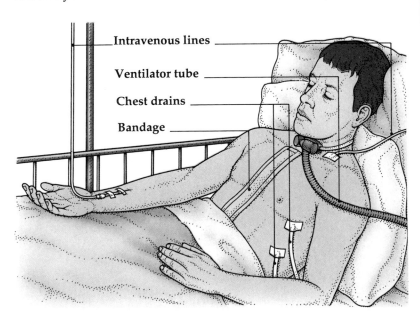

Intravenous lines

Ventilator tube

Chest drains

Bandage

ASK YOUR DOCTOR
LUNG TISSUE DISORDERS

Q My son's doctor says he has sarcoidosis, but my son is not being treated. Why not?

A Most people with sarcoidosis do not receive treatment because, in the early stages, the condition often improves by itself. If no improvement occurs, doctors prescribe corticosteroid drugs that treat inflammation, but these medications sometimes do not cure the disease. Your son's doctor will monitor his condition closely before deciding whether to treat him.

Q My mother has been taking an antibiotic for a urinary tract infection, but her doctor discontinued its use after she developed shortness of breath. She got better soon after. What happened?

A In rare cases, an antibacterial drug called nitrofurantoin can cause short-term inflammation of lung tissue. Fever, difficulty breathing, and coughing can appear from 2 hours to 10 days after the person begins taking the drug; these symptoms go away when use of the drug is discontinued. The cause of the reaction is unknown.

Q I have rheumatoid arthritis and my doctor says it has affected my lungs. How can a disease in my joints spread to my lungs?

A Rheumatoid arthritis is a systemic disease (one that affects your whole system) so it can affect any part of the body. The disorder can cause inflammation and scarring in the lungs. If your rheumatoid arthritis subsides, your lung condition should improve too.

LUNG CANCER

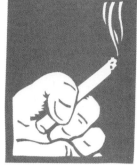

EACH YEAR ABOUT 150,000 Americans die of lung cancer, the most common type of cancer in both men and women. Overwhelming evidence shows that tobacco smoking causes about 90 percent of all cases. Thousands of lives would be saved every year if people stopped smoking. In rare instances, other causes of lung cancer have been cited, such as the inhalation of asbestos fibers by shipyard workers or the inhalation of radon gas by uranium miners.

The most common site at which lung cancer develops is inside a bronchus. Doctors call lung cancer that develops in a bronchus bronchogenic carcinoma. This type of lung cancer accounts for about 95 percent of all cases. Cancerous growths can also occur in other tissues inside the chest, including the pleural membranes that surround the lungs.

Cancer inside a bronchus can produce serious symptoms because the tumor blocks the passage of air into the person's lungs. Like all cancer, bronchogenic carcinoma causes disability and death by spreading to other parts of the body, by way of the bloodstream and lymph system. At the new site, the cancer invades more tissue.

SYMPTOMS OF BRONCHOGENIC CARCINOMA

An early symptom of lung cancer is a persistent or unusual kind of cough. An example of a late symptom is severe weight loss.

Early symptoms
Early symptoms, caused by the initial (primary) tumor, can include cough, phlegm, blood in the phlegm, and wheezing. Later, the person experiences breathlessness, chest pain, or fever.

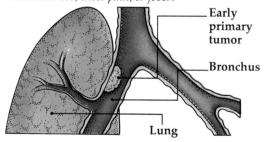

Early primary tumor

Bronchus

Lung

Later symptoms
Later symptoms arise from growth of the tumor, which can obstruct the flow of blood, air, or food. Symptoms include pain and difficulty swallowing.

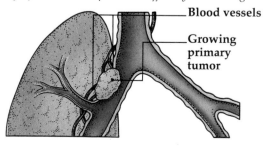

Blood vessels

Growing primary tumor

Symptoms of spreading cancer
When the tumor spreads to other sites, such as lymph nodes, bones, the brain, and the liver, doctors say the tumor has metastasized. Cancerous tissue that forms at the new site is called a metastasis. Symptoms include pain and loss of function in the affected areas. For example, paralysis may occur from loss of normal brain function or a weakened bone may fracture.

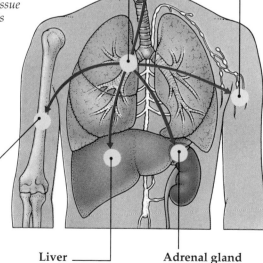

Brain metastasis

Primary tumor

Lymph node metastasis

Bone metastasis

Liver metastasis

Adrenal gland metastasis

Other symptoms
In a small number of people with lung cancer, symptoms develop that are not directly caused by the primary tumor or by a spreading tumor. These symptoms can include nervous system problems causing unsteadiness and muscle paralysis, arthritis, and rashes. Their exact cause is unknown.

TYPES OF BRONCHOGENIC CARCINOMA

The cells shown below were taken from the bronchi of people with lung cancer. They represent different types of bronchogenic carcinoma.

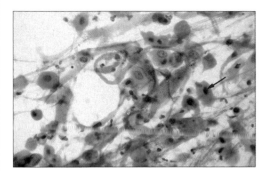

Squamous cell carcinoma

Squamous cell carcinoma (shown at left, magnified 460 times) accounts for about 30 to 40 percent of bronchogenic carcinomas. It is strongly linked to tobacco smoking and occurs mainly in the larger bronchi, where it can bleed and interfere with air flow. These tumors grow slowly. Most respond well to radiation therapy at first, but not to chemotherapy.

Small-cell carcinoma

Small-cell carcinoma (shown at right, magnified 400 times) accounts for 20 to 30 percent of bronchogenic carcinomas. Tobacco smoking is the probable cause. Tumors occur mainly in the major bronchi and can block air flow. The cancer spreads rapidly and extensively throughout the person's body. If treated early, it responds fairly well to chemotherapy, which may be combined with radiation therapy.

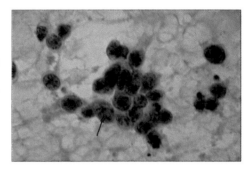

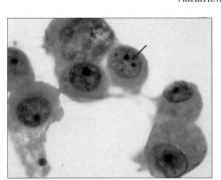

Large-cell carcinoma

Large-cell carcinoma (shown at left, magnified 360 times) accounts for 10 to 20 percent of bronchogenic carcinomas and is also strongly linked to tobacco smoking. Tumors can spread inside the lungs, to other structures in the chest cavity, and throughout the body. Chemotherapy and radiation therapy are usually ineffective.

Adenocarcinoma

Adenocarcinoma (shown at right, magnified 430 times) accounts for about 25 percent of bronchogenic carcinomas. Its link to tobacco use is less clear. Adenocarcinoma of a bronchus often spreads outside the chest cavity, primarily to the brain and spine. Adenocarcinoma affecting the lung's air sacs and/or the smallest airways can spread to large areas of lung tissue. These carcinomas do not respond well to chemotherapy, and radiation therapy is only partially effective.

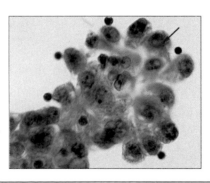

SECONDARY LUNG TUMORS

Cancer that starts in other parts of the body often spreads to the lungs by way of the bloodstream. Doctors refer to this type of lung cancer as a secondary lung tumor. The secondary tumor can cause symptoms such as shortness of breath and a cough. But the original, or primary, cancer often produces symptoms long before the lung cancer is diagnosed. Treatment varies, depending on the original site of the cancer. Doctors cannot treat spreading cancer by surgically removing it. Cancers that originate in the breast, bone, thyroid gland, and kidney are the most common cancers that spread to the lungs.

THE DOCTOR'S INVESTIGATIONS

The doctor's examination may reveal no evidence of disease. But sometimes the doctor detects abnormal breathing sounds caused by a tumor obstructing an airway. He or she may also find signs of pneumonia or pleural effusion (see page 89). In other cases, the doctor finds hardened, enlarged lymph glands in the person's neck or armpit, an enlarged liver, or signs of impaired brain or nerve function. Such findings indicate that the cancer has spread to sites in the body outside the person's lung. To reach a diagnosis, the doctor orders tests.

Results of imaging techniques

If a cancer is present in the lung, a chest X-ray will usually reveal it. In some cases, complicating factors produced by the cancer, such as pleural effusion (see page 89), pneumonia, lymph node enlargement, or lung collapse, may obscure the cancer. The doctor may be able to see these signs, but not the tumor itself.

If the doctor sees an abnormality on the chest X-ray, a computed tomography (CT) scan of the chest may be performed. The CT scan shows any spread of the cancer to the lymph nodes that may not have been detected on the chest X-ray. Doctors often order CT scans of the brain, liver, and adrenal glands, common sites to which cancer spreads.

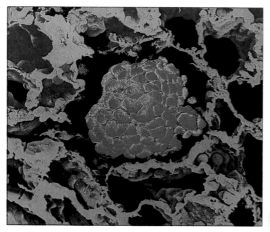

Cancer cells in the lung
A doctor may perform a bronchoscopy (see page 80) to obtain samples of tissue or bronchial secretions. The photograph above (magnified 320 times) shows cancer cells (red area) in lung tissue. A number of cancer cells have separated from the main mass.

Confirming the diagnosis

The doctor can confirm the diagnosis by looking at cancerous cells from the tumor under a microscope. Doctors obtain these cells from samples of lung or bronchial secretions or tissue (see above). If fluid has accumulated between the pleural membranes, which surround the lungs, the doctor may obtain samples of both fluid and pleural tissue (see PLEURAL AND LUNG BIOPSIES on page 81) to identify any cancer cells present.

THE DECISION TO OPERATE

Once doctors confirm a diagnosis of cancer, they must decide whether to recommend surgery. If the cancer has spread outside the person's lungs, lung surgery will not be of benefit. Most people with lung cancer are or have been smokers and often have another lung disease, such as emphysema. The doctor may perform tests of lung function (see below) to find out whether the person would be able to breathe with the lung tissue remaining after surgery without the help of oxygen or a ventilator. If the person could not breathe without help, surgery would not be performed.

Testing lung function
To test how well a person's lungs are functioning, doctors measure the forced expiratory volume in 1 second (FEV_1) – the maximum volume of air the person can breathe out forcibly in 1 second. The graphs below compare the volume of air forcibly exhaled by a person with healthy lungs (upper graph) to the reduced volume exhaled by a heavy smoker. Doctors sometimes use this test to find out whether a person with lung disease can tolerate extensive lung surgery.

Normal lung function

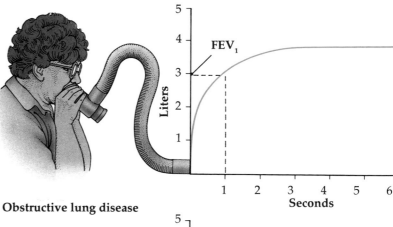

Obstructive lung disease

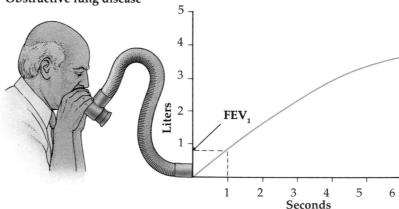

CANCER OF THE PLEURA

A tumor of the membranes that surround the lungs is called mesothelioma. It can cause severe chest pain, coughing, and difficulty breathing. The tumor may cause no symptoms until it becomes large. Its incidence is high in people who have been exposed to asbestos fibers. Mesothelioma is incurable. It does not respond well to surgery, radiation therapy, or chemotherapy.

SURGICAL PROCEDURES
LOBECTOMY FOR LUNG CANCER

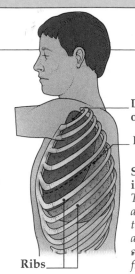

ONLY ABOUT 5 TO 10 PERCENT **of people who have lung cancer can be completely cured by surgery, but about 25 to 30 percent can be helped by surgery. Removal of a lobe of the lung (lobectomy) is successful only if the person can breathe unassisted with the remaining lung tissue. The cancer must also be limited to a specific area, with no evidence of spread to other parts of the body.**

Diseased lobe of lung

Incision

Site of the incision
The surgeon makes an incision around the side of the chest, along the line of the space between the fifth and sixth ribs.

Ribs

1 Before surgery, the person receives tranquilizing drugs and a general anesthetic. The surgeon makes an incision through the skin around the side of the person's chest and cuts the muscles between the ribs. The surgeon spreads the ribs apart to reveal the lung with its thin covering, the pleura.

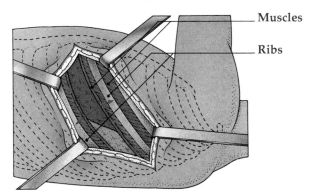

Muscles

Ribs

3 The surgeon ties off and then cuts the arteries, veins, and bronchus supplying the affected lobe. After closing off the stump of the bronchus to prevent air leakage, the surgeon removes the diseased lobe.

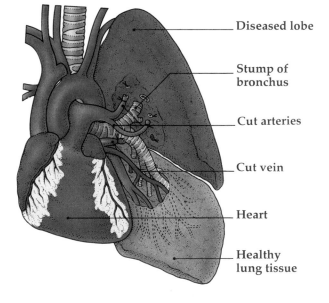

Diseased lobe

Stump of bronchus

Cut arteries

Cut vein

Heart

Healthy lung tissue

2 The surgeon moves the affected lobe aside to expose lymph nodes and blood vessels and takes samples from the lymph nodes. These samples are examined under a microscope to find out whether the cancer has spread.

Diseased lobe

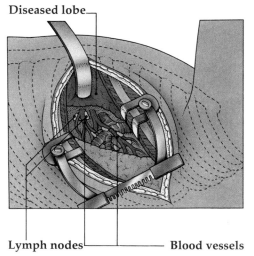

Lymph nodes   Blood vessels

4 The surgeon inserts two drains into the back part of the chest before sewing up the incision. These drain excess blood and fluid from around the lungs and remove any air that leaks into the chest cavity. The drains are removed 3 to 5 days later. The person usually leaves the hospital in about 10 days.

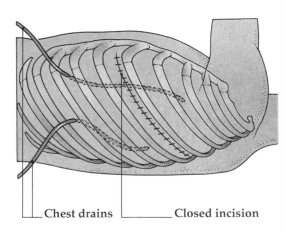

Chest drains   Closed incision

ASK YOUR DOCTOR
LUNG CANCER

Q **Recently, I have been coughing up blood, which really scares me. Could I have lung cancer?**

A Although coughing up blood can be a sign of lung cancer, cancer is not the only possible cause. Other causes include bronchitis accompanied by a raspy cough (which bruises tiny vessels in the lining of the bronchi), a severe chest infection, or blood clots lodged in a lung. See your doctor immediately. If you do have lung cancer, early diagnosis and treatment give you the best chance of survival. If you don't have cancer, your doctor may still want to treat your condition.

Q **My mother died of lung cancer. Is lung cancer hereditary? Can my children and I do anything to avoid it?**

A In extremely rare cases, lung cancer can be hereditary. But lung cancer is much more common in people who smoke cigarettes, regardless of their family history. The most important thing you can do is to avoid smoking and to tell your children not to smoke.

Q **I had pneumonia a few months ago. It cleared up, but now it's back again. I've read that lung cancer can cause pneumonia-like symptoms. Is this true?**

A Sometimes pneumonia recurs or becomes chronic (long-term) and does not go away. In rare cases, a tumor can partially block a bronchus, causing pneumonia. See your doctor. He or she will perform a chest X-ray and a CT scan and will take phlegm samples to reach the correct diagnosis of your condition.

TREATMENT

Surgical removal of a lung cancer offers the only chance of complete cure. Surgery is possible only if the cancer has not spread to other parts of the body. During surgery, the cancer and surrounding lung tissue are removed. In rare cases, if the cancer has spread up the main bronchus that supplies the affected lung, surgeons may remove the entire lung on that side.

Small-cell carcinoma sometimes responds to chemotherapy, which can help prolong the survival of people with this rapidly spreading type of cancer. But for most types of lung cancer, the results of chemotherapy have been disappointing. Chemotherapy also causes unpleasant side effects, such as hair loss, fatigue, aching, nausea, infection, and anemia.

OUTLOOK FOR LUNG CANCER

The outlook for people with lung cancer is poor. Even people whose tumors have not spread usually die within 5 years after the diagnosis. Only those who have a very small tumor that is limited to a small area near the surface of the lung and who have it removed surgically have a good chance of being alive in 5 years. The message is clear: to avoid getting lung cancer, do not smoke.

Radiation therapy
If doctors consider a person's lung cancer inoperable, they may give the person radiation therapy, which helps shrink the tumor and alleviate some symptoms. Beams of radiation strike the tumor from different angles (see upper illustration below) to ensure that the tumor receives a higher dose of radiation than the surrounding tissues (see lower illustration below).

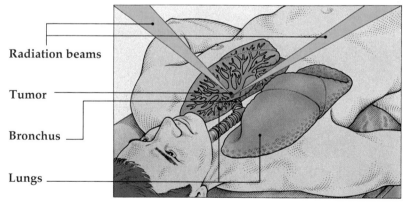

Radiation beams

Tumor

Bronchus

Lungs

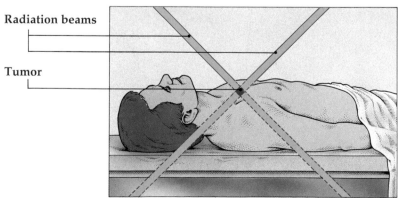

Radiation beams

Tumor

CASE HISTORY
COUGHING UP BLOOD

EVE HAS SMOKED a pack of cigarettes a day since she was a teenager and has had a persistent smokers' cough for many years. The cough has always been especially bad when she first wakes up but seems to be relieved by her first cigarette. One morning, Eve became alarmed when she coughed up phlegm streaked with bright red blood. She made an appointment to see her doctor that day.

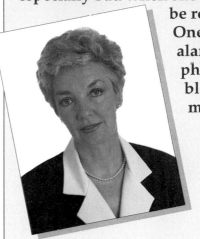

PERSONAL DETAILS
Name Eve Brown
Age 54
Occupation Executive secretary
Family Father was an alcoholic who died after a stroke. Mother is healthy, except for arthritis.

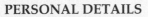

Eve's chest X-ray
The doctor sees a round white area (arrow) on Eve's chest X-ray that he suspects could be a tumor. Additional tests confirm that the tumor is cancerous.

THE OUTCOME

About a year after her operation, Eve develops a severe backache and tender nodules in her skin. Examination by her doctor shows that both symptoms are caused by the growth of cancerous tumors. These tumors must have developed from cancer cells that spread from the lung to other parts of her body but were too small to have been detected by the CT scan. The doctor tells Eve that radiation therapy and chemotherapy can relieve her symptoms. After treatment, her backache and skin nodules improve. But another tumor is found in Eve's chest. She develops pneumonia and dies a week later.

MEDICAL BACKGROUND

Aside from her persistent cough, Eve feels fine and has had no major illnesses. She is overweight and occasionally diets. She has recently lost 12 pounds without really trying.

THE INITIAL CONSULTATION

The doctor's examination shows no evidence of disease, but the weight loss and coughing up of blood make the doctor suspicious. Eve's doctor refers her to a lung specialist.

THE SPECIALIST'S CONSULTATION

The specialist orders a chest X-ray, which shows a round opaque area in the middle of Eve's chest on the right side that could be a tumor. A sample of Eve's bronchial mucus shows no evidence of cancerous cells. The specialist performs fiberoptic bronchoscopy (examination with a viewing tube) to obtain tissue from the lining of her right bronchus. The doctor sends the tissue to the laboratory for examination and analysis.

THE DIAGNOSIS AND TREATMENT

The test result confirms SQUAMOUS CELL CARCINOMA (lung cancer). A computed tomography (CT) scan shows no evidence that the growth has spread, and the results of tests of Eve's lung function are normal, indicating that her cancer can be treated by removing the tumor.

Eve has surgery to remove the diseased lung tissue. She recovers well from her operation and returns to work after several months.

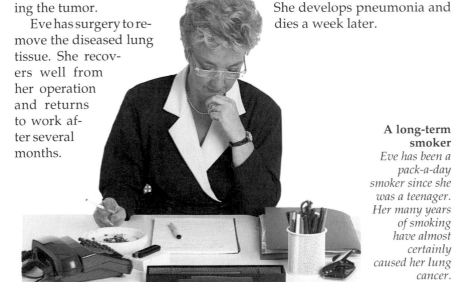

A long-term smoker
Eve has been a pack-a-day smoker since she was a teenager. Her many years of smoking have almost certainly caused her lung cancer.

129

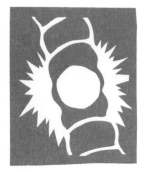

INHALED OBJECTS

AN OBJECT THAT YOU accidentally inhale may become stuck in an airway. If you cannot cough it out and it lodges in your trachea, it could cut off your air supply and you would need emergency treatment. Sometimes an inhaled object passes farther down the respiratory tract and lodges in a small airway in the lungs. When this happens, the object does not interfere with breathing but can eventually cause pneumonia or a lung abscess.

Choking is the sixth most common cause of accidental death. In 1989, an estimated 3,900 people in the US suffocated after food or another object blocked an airway. Children under 4 years, who can choke on almost any small object, and older people are especially at risk.

In adults, the most common cause of choking is a piece of food that lodges in the person's larynx. This type of choking occurs more commonly in people who have been drinking alcohol.

SYMPTOMS

Partial obstruction of an airway by an inhaled object causes coughing, noisy, labored breathing, and, if the vocal cords have been irritated, hoarseness. Obstruction often occurs when a child throws food into the air and attempts to catch it in his or her mouth. The piece of food can fall down the child's throat, be inhaled, and lodge in a bronchus or a smaller airway in the child's lung. Coughing usually dislodges the object. Complete obstruction of the larynx is a life-threatening emergency. If the person is not treated immediately, he or she can die within a few minutes. A person who is suffocating will show obvious signs of distress, grasp his or her neck, and make strenuous but ineffective efforts to breathe. His or her face turns red and then purple. The most effective treatment for choking is the Heimlich maneuver (see right), which even an untrained person can perform on the spot.

WARNING

A small object can become lodged in a bronchus or can pass down into the small airways of the lung. Coughing and choking eventually subside, and there is often no immediate indication that anything is wrong. But if the object is not removed promptly, it can cause a lung abscess or lung collapse. Call a doctor immediately if you suspect that you have inhaled a small object (or that someone else has).

PERFORMING THE HEIMLICH MANEUVER

This procedure uses a rapid upward thrust from below the breastbone to push the diaphragm up and forcefully expel air and the obstructing object from the person's mouth. Use the Heimlich maneuver only if the person is conscious.

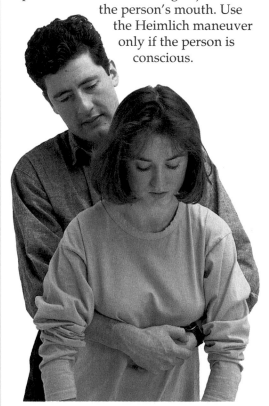

For an adult
Stand behind the person and place your arms around his or her waist. Place your fist just below the angle between the ribs with the thumb side against the person's stomach. Grip your fist with your other hand and thrust your fist up and in, quickly and forcefully, four times. Do not squeeze the person's ribs with your arms. You may need to repeat the maneuver six to 10 times.

FIRST AID FOR CHOKING

The best first-aid procedure for someone who is choking is the Heimlich maneuver. If this maneuver fails, call an ambulance immediately. The trained rescuer may perform a cricothyrotomy – an emergency procedure in which an opening is made in the trachea, and a tube is inserted to bypass the obstruction.

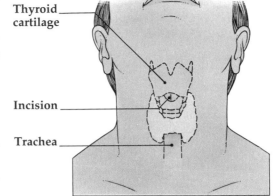

Thyroid cartilage

Incision

Trachea

Cricothyrotomy
A doctor or a trained rescuer makes a vertical cut in the middle of the person's neck just below the lower edge of the Adam's apple (the thyroid cartilage). A small metal or plastic tube placed in the trachea keeps it open until the inhaled object can be removed.

INVESTIGATION AND REMOVAL

X-ray examination may show an inhaled object or collapse of part of the lung, indicating that an object may be blocking an airway. Doctors can usually remove the inhaled object with a bronchoscope (see below).

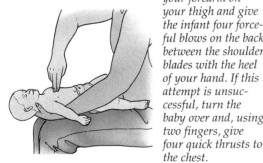

For a child
Perform the Heimlich maneuver in the same way as you would for an adult, but using slightly less pressure. You may need to lift the child off the ground.

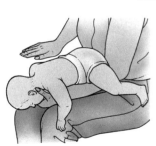

For an infant
Place the infant face down across your forearm. Make sure the baby's head is lower than his or her chest. Support the head by firmly holding the jaw. Rest your forearm on your thigh and give the infant four forceful blows on the back between the shoulder blades with the heel of your hand. If this attempt is unsuccessful, turn the baby over and, using two fingers, give four quick thrusts to the chest.

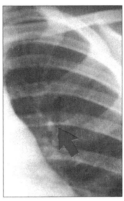

X-ray of an inhaled object
This X-ray shows the area in which the inhaled object has lodged (arrow) in the left main bronchus of a child.

Bronchoscopy
The doctor inserts a bronchoscope, a tubelike viewing instrument, through the person's mouth and into the airway, to examine the inside of the bronchi. Once the doctor locates the inhaled object, he or she can remove it with forceps that the doctor inserts through the bronchoscope.

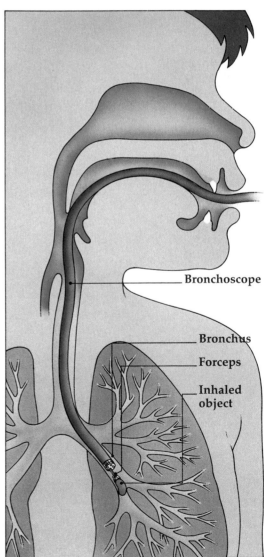

Bronchoscope

Bronchus

Forceps

Inhaled object

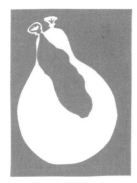

PNEUMOTHORAX AND LUNG COLLAPSE

ADOUBLE-LAYERED MEMBRANE called the pleura surrounds your lungs and covers your inner chest wall. It keeps the chest cavity airtight. If air enters the space between the two layers of the pleura, a condition known as pneumothorax occurs, which causes a collapse of the lung. Blockage of the air passages to the lungs causes another type of lung collapse called atelectasis.

What happens in a pneumothorax?
Both your lungs and your chest wall are elastic and pull in opposite directions, causing a delicate balance of opposing pressures between the pleural membranes. This balance enables the lungs to inflate. If air enters the pleural space, it upsets the balance between the pleural membranes. The lung collapses inward and the chest wall springs outward.

HEALTHY LUNGS

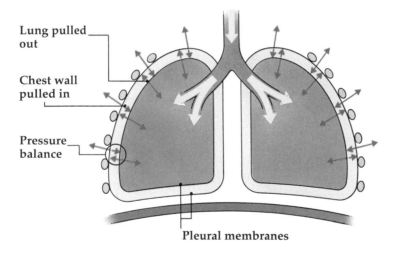

Lung pulled out

Chest wall pulled in

Pressure balance

Pleural membranes

PNEUMOTHORAX

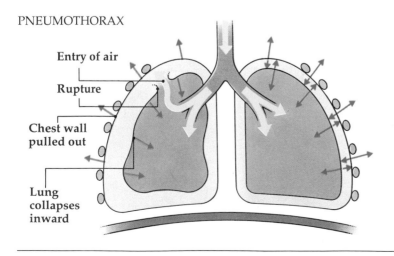

Entry of air

Rupture

Chest wall pulled out

Lung collapses inward

The pleural layer that adheres directly to each lung is called the visceral pleura. Another pleural membrane, the parietal pleura, adheres to the inside of your chest wall. A thin, lubricating film that lies between the two layers allows them to slide against each other easily when your lungs inflate each time you breathe.

PNEUMOTHORAX

When a pleural membrane ruptures, air can enter the pleural space, causing the lung to collapse. No air can move into or out of the collapsed part of the lung, and the exchange of oxygen and carbon dioxide cannot take place.

Types of pneumothorax

In a spontaneous pneumothorax, air passes from the lung into the pleural space by way of a rupture in the pleura next to the lung. The causes are not fully understood, but doctors think the ruptures occur at weak spots (called blebs) in the pleura, usually near the top of the lung. Spontaneous pneumothorax can also occur in people with underlying lung disorders, such as emphysema, tuberculosis, a lung abscess, or cystic fibrosis. Spontaneous pneumothorax occurs six times more often in men than in women because men more commonly contract these underlying lung diseases. For unknown reasons, affected people are often young, tall, and thin. Once a

DRAINING A PNEUMOTHORAX

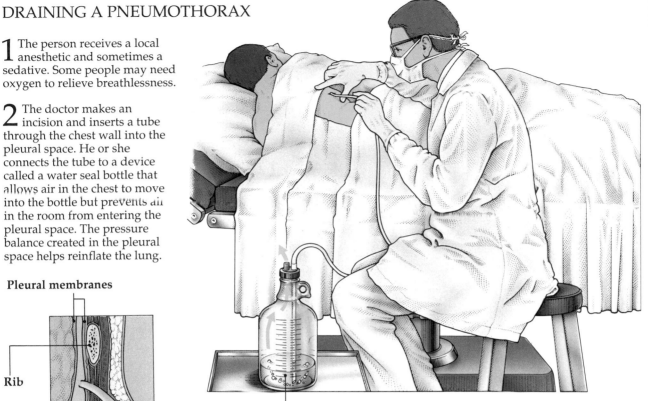

1 The person receives a local anesthetic and sometimes a sedative. Some people may need oxygen to relieve breathlessness.

2 The doctor makes an incision and inserts a tube through the chest wall into the pleural space. He or she connects the tube to a device called a water seal bottle that allows air in the chest to move into the bottle but prevents air in the room from entering the pleural space. The pressure balance created in the pleural space helps reinflate the lung.

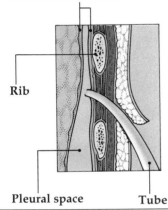

Pleural membranes

Rib

Pleural space　　**Tube**

Water seal bottle

3 When air from the pleural space enters the water seal bottle, it makes the water in the bottle bubble. The doctor knows the leak has stopped when the water in the water seal bottle stops bubbling. The doctor may remove the tube during the next day or two and will cover the incision with a dressing.

person has had a spontaneous pneumothorax, he or she risks a recurrence within an average of 2 years.

Penetrating wounds to the chest can also cause air to enter the pleura, leading to lung collapse. Such wounds result from injuries caused by sharp instruments such as knives, from accidents in which broken ribs penetrate the pleura, or from invasive medical procedures, such as a lung biopsy (see page 81). Air can enter the pleural space from outside the chest or from inside the lung.

Symptoms, diagnosis, and treatment

People with a pneumothorax experience chest pain, which often develops abruptly at rest, and breathlessness, which may become progressively worse. The pain is confined to the side on which the lung has collapsed. People with a pneumothorax caused by lung disease often have more breathing difficulty because their lungs already function poorly.

To diagnose a pneumothorax, doctors observe and feel the person's chest to see whether the affected side moves less than usual during breathing. Pneumothorax causes the lungs' natural "muffling" effect to be lost, allowing the air in the chest to resonate. The doctor will tap the person's chest to listen for increased resonance. The doctor listens for diminished or absent breath sounds over the area of the collapse and confirms the diagnosis by a chest X-ray. If a pneumothorax has occurred, the X-ray will show that the edge of the lung has moved away from the chest wall.

TENSION PNEUMOTHORAX

Tension pneumothorax occurs when air that has entered the pleural space cannot escape and begins to accumulate. The pressure in the pleural space increases and can compress the healthy lung and heart. This process can lead to a potentially life-threatening emergency. To treat the condition, doctors remove the accumulated air (see DRAINING A PNEUMOTHORAX, above).

The separation between the lung and chest wall is more apparent if the person exhales fully before the X-ray.

Treatment of a pneumothorax depends on the amount of air in the chest, the extent of the collapse, and the presence of other disease. A small pneumothorax may not need treatment. Doctors treat others by sucking the air out with a needle and syringe. Doctors drain most pneumothoraces with a chest tube and a water seal bottle (see page 133). If the pneumothorax recurs, doctors introduce an irritant that causes an inflammation, making the two pleural membranes fuse together as they heal. Surgery may also be considered. During the operation, the surgeon either scrapes the surface of the pleura to provoke scar formation, causing its two layers to stick together, or cuts out the area of lung that has ruptured.

ATELECTASIS

In the type of lung collapse called atelectasis, the cause of the collapse is obstruction of either the air passages of the lungs or a pulmonary artery. Airway obstruction can result from a plug of dry mucus, from an object accidentally inhaled, or from a tumor.

There may be few or no symptoms of a small lung collapse. But some large lung collapses cause definite breathlessness and anxiety. Other symptoms depend on possible underlying disease.

Investigation and treatment

A chest X-ray helps the doctor diagnose a lung collapse. Doctors use other tests to help them diagnose an underlying disease that might have caused the person's lung to collapse. Treatment depends on the cause of the lung collapse. It may include postural drainage (see page 121), or bronchoscopy (see page 80) to remove a plug of mucus or an inhaled object, antibiotics if an infection is present, or radiation therapy to shrink an obstructing tumor.

INVESTIGATING LUNG COLLAPSE

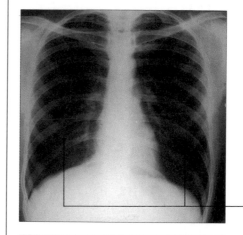

What the X-rays reveal
The chest X-ray at left shows two healthy lungs. The X-ray at lower left reveals a complete collapse of the right lung (left side of image). No air can enter the collapsed lung, and it becomes a solid, dense mass that appears as a white area on the X-ray.

Normal lungs

Collapsed lung

Normal lung

What happens when a lung collapses?
When an airway supplying the lung becomes blocked, the blockage acts like a valve that allows air out but does not allow air in. The air-deprived portion of lung becomes solid and compressed.

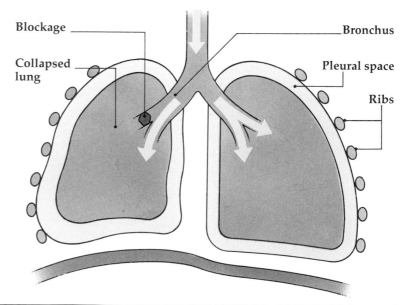

Blockage

Collapsed lung

Bronchus

Pleural space

Ribs

CASE HISTORY
SUDDEN CHEST PAIN AND BREATHLESSNESS

THREE YEARS AGO, Brian had a spontaneous pneumothorax (air between the two membranes surrounding his lungs). The doctors removed the air but told Brian that the pneumothorax could recur. When Brian again began having sudden, severe chest pain and breathlessness, he asked his neighbor to drive him to his doctor's office right away.

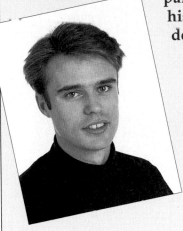

PERSONAL DETAILS
Name Brian Nordstrom
Age 23
Occupation Salesperson
Family Parents and two sisters are healthy. No family history of lung-related disease.

MEDICAL BACKGROUND
Brian is physically fit and healthy. He does not smoke and has had no major illnesses. He broke his arm last year when he went skiing but has recovered completely.

THE CONSULTATION
By the time Brian arrives at his doctor's office, he is so breathless that he can hardly speak. The doctor immediately notices a bluish tinge to Brian's lips and fingernails and can see that there is less movement of Brian's chest on the right side than on the left. Percussion (tapping) of the chest shows that the right side is unusually resonant. Listening with a stethoscope, the doctor hears diminished breath sounds in the upper part of Brian's right lung. The doctor prescribes painkillers and sends Brian for chest X-rays.

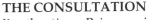

The doctor's examination
The doctor hears diminished breath sounds coming from the upper right part of Brian's chest.

THE DIAGNOSIS
The chest X-rays show a black, air-filled area on the right side of Brian's chest and that his heart has shifted to the left. His shrunken right lung has a small blisterlike opening on its surface. The doctor tells Brian that he has had another SPONTANEOUS PNEUMOTHORAX and that if the blister does not close, the portion of lung on which it lies will have to be removed. The doctor explains that this condition usually occurs for no apparent reason and often strikes thin, young men – like Brian – who have no underlying disease.

THE TREATMENT
Brian is rushed to the hospital where doctors insert a small drain into his chest and try four times to remove the air. Every time they disconnect the drain, the lung collapses. The doctors tell Brian that they must perform surgery because the blister will not heal. Brian agrees. He is taken to the operating room, where doctors remove a small wedge-shaped portion of lung.

Brian makes a steady recovery and, after 10 days, he goes home from the hospital. The doctor tells Brian that he can return to work in about 2 weeks or whenever he feels ready. The doctor also tells Brian he can take a mild painkiller, such as acetaminophen, if he needs one.

THE OUTCOME
Brian quickly improves. The doctor tells him that, because the surgeons removed the weakened area of his lung, he should not experience any more episodes of spontaneous pneumothorax.

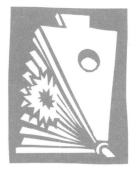

RESPIRATORY DISTRESS AND FAILURE

CAUSED BY A VARIETY of disorders, respiratory distress and respiratory failure are serious conditions that severely restrict the ability to breathe. This restriction of breathing impairs the transport of vital oxygen to and the removal of carbon dioxide from the cells of your body.

Treatment for respiratory failure
Bronchodilator drugs, which a person takes through an inhaler, help open the airways. These drugs are also used to treat asthma, which can be an underlying cause of respiratory failure.

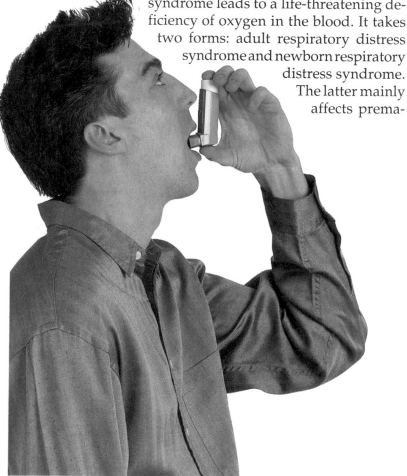

When a person experiences respiratory failure, the level of oxygen in his or her blood is too low and the level of carbon dioxide is too high. Respiratory failure can arise from diseases that affect the lungs or from diseases that affect other parts of the body; for example, when muscle paralysis prevents the lungs from doing their job. Respiratory distress syndrome leads to a life-threatening deficiency of oxygen in the blood. It takes two forms: adult respiratory distress syndrome and newborn respiratory distress syndrome. The latter mainly affects prema-ture infants who, because their lungs are not mature, cannot maintain the breathing process.

RESPIRATORY FAILURE

Any condition that disrupts the normal exchange of oxygen and carbon dioxide in the lungs can result in respiratory failure. The underlying condition is often a lung disorder, such as chronic bronchitis, emphysema (especially if accompanied by a chest infection), pneumonia, pulmonary edema (fluid in the lungs), or severe asthma. But other conditions, including a drug overdose, can also cause respiratory failure.

Diagnosis and treatment
The signs of respiratory failure that doctors look for include cyanosis (blue discoloration of the lips and nails) and confusion. The person's breathing rate may increase or decrease depending on the cause. Doctors confirm the diagnosis by a test that shows whether the levels of oxygen and carbon dioxide in the person's blood are abnormal.

Most people with respiratory failure need oxygen to raise the level of this gas in the blood. Further treatment depends on the underlying disorder. For example, doctors prescribe antibiotics to treat chest infections. In severe cases, the person may need mechanical assistance with breathing, especially when carbon dioxide levels in the blood are high.

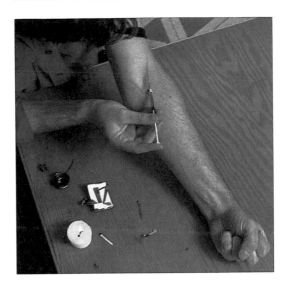

**A cause of respiratory
failure in a person with healthy lungs**
An overdose of narcotic drugs can cause respiratory failure by producing an accumulation of fluid in the air sacs in the lungs or by suppressing the respiratory center in the brain.

ADULT RESPIRATORY DISTRESS SYNDROME

Adult respiratory distress syndrome is a serious condition that usually leads to respiratory failure. It develops in some people whose lungs have been damaged by disease or injury. The lung tissue becomes so stiff it cannot expand and becomes filled with fluid. Possible causes of adult respiratory distress syndrome include severe pneumonia, near drowning, drug overdose, inhalation of vomit, and inhalation of an irritant gas, such as chlorine. The condition can also occur after a serious illness, such as septicemia (poisoning of the blood by bacteria). Because respiratory distress syndrome can develop after a severe injury, it is sometimes called "shock lung."

Symptoms include an increased breathing rate and breathlessness. As the condition progresses, the person may turn blue and, unless treated, will die.

Diagnosis and treatment
Doctors diagnose adult respiratory distress syndrome by physical examination and tests, such as an analysis of the levels of oxygen and carbon dioxide in the person's blood and chest X-rays. Affected people must receive treatment in the intensive care unit of a hospital. The person receives oxygen, but if his or her condition is very serious or if it deteriorates, the doctor will order mechanical ventilation until the person can breathe without help. Doctors often give corticosteroid drugs (see page 96), delivered intravenously, and antibiotics. The overall survival rate for people with respiratory distress syndrome is about 50 percent. Some people who survive have permanent lung damage.

"Shock lung"
Adult respiratory distress syndrome can develop after a serious injury, such as occurs in a traffic accident. The condition usually does not become obvious for 24 to 72 hours after the initial trauma.

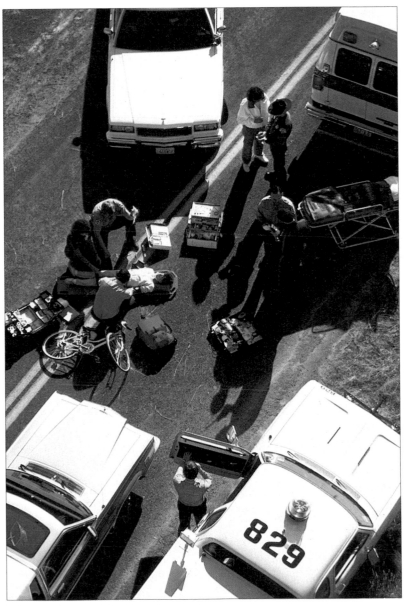

ARTIFICIAL VENTILATION

When respiratory distress or respiratory failure develops, a person may no longer be able to breathe on his or her own. Doctors can save the person's life only if breathing is performed artificially. For a short time, artificial ventilation can be performed by mouth-to-mouth resuscitation. But for periods of hours or longer, the person needs help from a mechanical device. Mechanical ventilators pump air into the lungs through a tube inserted into the person's windpipe. Today's computerized machines control the amount of air the person receives, the rate at which it flows, and the pressure exerted on the person's airways.

Doctors regularly check the levels of oxygen and carbon dioxide in the blood of a person who is breathing with a ventilator to ensure that the levels remain normal. They also monitor the person's blood pressure and temperature. People receiving artificial ventilation cannot eat or drink, so nutrients are given through a tube inserted into the person's mouth that extends into the stomach. The person receives medications through a needle inserted into his or her vein.

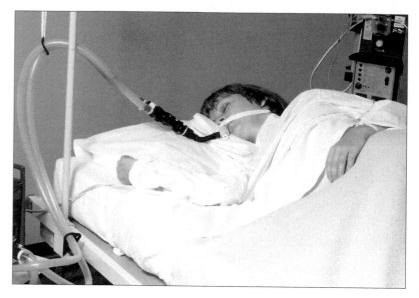

Breathing with the help of a ventilator
The machine pumps air through a tube (called an endotracheal tube) that is inserted into the person's windpipe through the mouth or nose or through an artificial opening created in the front of the person's neck (a tracheostomy).

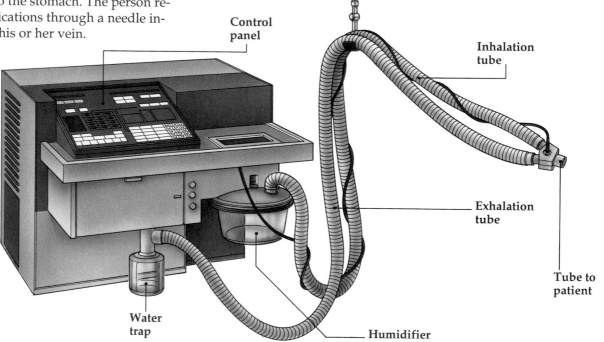

Control panel

Inhalation tube

Exhalation tube

Tube to patient

Water trap

Humidifier

How a ventilator works
Ventilators work by inflating the patient's lungs with air. Today's ventilators control such factors as the duration of each breath and the pressure applied to the person's airways to minimize the possibility of heart failure from unrestrained pressure that could compress the veins leading to the heart. The machine pumps the air through a humidifier before it reaches the person to prevent the person's lungs from drying out as air passes in or out. The oxygen content can be altered to suit each person's needs.

NEWBORN RESPIRATORY DISTRESS SYNDROME

Newborn respiratory distress syndrome can occur in premature infants whose lungs are not mature enough to function. The infant's underdeveloped lungs have a deficiency of surfactant, a substance that prevents the air sacs (alveoli) of the lungs from collapsing. Inhalation of vomit can cause this syndrome in a full-term newborn.

Doctors treat babies with newborn respiratory distress syndrome in a neonatal (newborn) intensive care unit. Doctors keep the oxygen in the baby's blood at a safe level, watch the oxygen and carbon dioxide levels closely, and have mechanical devices ready to take over the baby's breathing if needed. A new treatment for respiratory distress syndrome in premature babies uses surfactant from cow lungs, given through a breathing tube (see page 28).

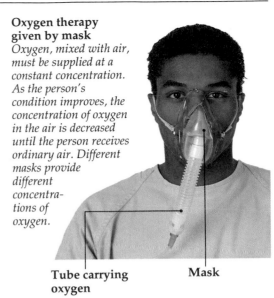

Oxygen therapy given by mask
Oxygen, mixed with air, must be supplied at a constant concentration. As the person's condition improves, the concentration of oxygen in the air is decreased until the person receives ordinary air. Different masks provide different concentrations of oxygen.

Tube carrying oxygen **Mask**

OXYGEN THERAPY

In both respiratory failure and adult respiratory distress syndrome, oxygen therapy must be provided to keep the amount of oxygen in the person's blood high enough to maintain the person's vital organs and sustain life. People can receive oxygen-enriched, humidified air continuously through a tube inserted into the nostrils or through a mask. The amount of oxygen and the rate at which it flows can be varied as needed.

Careful regulation

Oxygen therapy is often lifesaving but can produce problems. Pure oxygen, or oxygen in a very high concentration, is toxic if inhaled for more than a few hours. It causes bronchial irritation and may result in fluid in the lungs. Prolonged inhalation of oxygen in high concentrations can cause adult respiratory distress syndrome. In people who have emphysema, too much oxygen can suppress breathing rather than improve it. Doctors must regulate the concentration of oxygen supplied. It must be high enough to treat low oxygen levels in the blood but not so high that it suppresses breathing. Concentrations of oxygen greater than 50 percent are used only in critically ill persons.

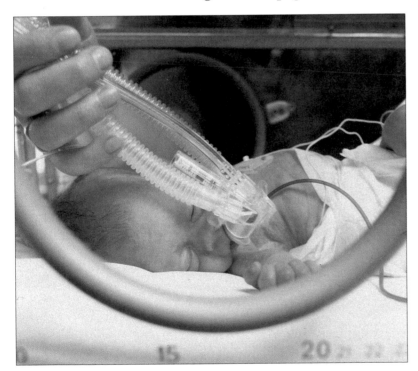

Continuous positive airway pressure
One way to ensure that a premature or newborn baby receives an adequate supply of oxygen is to use continuous positive airway pressure. This method steadily supplies oxygen-enriched air under slight pressure to the baby through a tube inserted into the baby's mouth.

GLOSSARY OF TERMS

Terms in *italics* refer to other terms listed in the glossary.

A

Adult respiratory distress syndrome
Any condition in adults that causes a life-threatening interference with the passage of oxygen from the air sacs in the lungs to the blood.

Allergic rhinitis
Inflammation of the mucous membrane that lines the nose caused by release of *histamine* and other substances that cause inflammation from *mast cells* following contact with an allergen.

Alpha₁-antitrypsin
A substance in the blood serum that neutralizes the action of certain enzymes released from white blood cells. When it is absent, these enzymes become active, destroy the *alveoli*, and cause *emphysema*.

Alveoli
The small air sacs contained in the lungs. Oxygen passes into the blood and carbon dioxide passes out of the blood through the walls of the alveoli.

Anaphylaxis
An unusually severe allergic reaction to a protein or other substance. The effects on the body may include breathing difficulty and can be fatal.

Anoxemia
The complete absence of oxygen in blood.

Anoxia
The complete absence of oxygen in a body tissue.

Antibody
A substance produced by the immune system that helps destroy invading microorganisms, proteins, or *antigens*.

Antigen
Anything that induces the body's immune system to respond by producing *antibodies*.

Apnea
Cessation of breathing.

Asphyxiation
The process by which a person stops breathing completely or receives inadequate oxygen in inhaled air. Asphyxiation can be caused by smothering, strangulation, drowning, or airway obstruction by an inhaled object or swelling of the lining of the larynx.

Aspiration pneumonia
Inflammation of lung tissues caused by inhaling irritating substances, such as vomited stomach acid.

Asthma
A disease characterized by cough, wheezing, shortness of breath, a sensation of chest tightness, and episodes of narrowing of segmental *bronchi* and *bronchioles*. The condition can result from allergy.

Atelectasis
Failure of a lung, or part of a lung, to expand at birth or the collapse of part or all of a lung that had been expanded normally. Collapse of lung tissue is most commonly caused by an obstruction in a *bronchus*.

Atopy
An inherited tendency to develop certain manifestations of allergy, such as *asthma* or the skin condition known as eczema.

B

Barotrauma
Damage or pain caused by a change in atmospheric pressure, often affecting the eardrums. Pressure developing during mechanical ventilation can produce a *pneumothorax*, another form of barotrauma.

Berylliosis
A rare occupational lung disease caused by inhaling dust or fumes of the metal beryllium.

Bleb
A space containing air, usually caused by the coalescence of *alveoli*, on the surface of the lung. The bleb can burst, causing a *pneumothorax*.

Bronchiole
One of the smaller branches of the segmental *bronchi* inside the lungs.

Bronchiolitis
A serious, life-threatening infection of the lungs, usually caused by a virus, mainly affecting babies and young children, in which inflammation of the *bronchioles* occurs.

Bronchitis
Inflammation of the *bronchi*, resulting in a cough, and occasionally a wheeze and shortness of breath, that produces large amounts of phlegm.

Bronchoconstriction
Narrowing of the airways caused by muscle contraction and/or mucous membrane congestion.

Bronchodilators
Drugs that widen constricted airways and improve breathing. Many such drugs are administered through an inhaler.

Bronchogenic carcinoma
The most common type of malignant (cancerous) lung tumor. The tumor usually develops in the lining of one of the main *bronchi* or larger *bronchioles*.

Bronchopneumonia
The most common form of *pneumonia* in which the inflammation spreads throughout the lung in small patches. It often causes death in bedridden, chronically ill patients.

Bronchoscopy
Examination of the main airways of the lungs by means of a hollow rigid or flexible fiberoptic endoscope (tube).

Bronchus
One of the main air passages that enter the lungs. The right main bronchus and the left main bronchus originate at the end of the *trachea* and branch into progressively smaller airways, ending in the *alveoli*.

C–F

Chronic obstructive pulmonary disease
Chronic *bronchitis* and/or *emphysema* that causes limitation of airflow.

Cricothyrotomy
Emergency surgery that creates an opening in the trachea so a person with an obstructed airway can breathe.

Cyanosis
Bluish coloration of the skin and mucous membranes caused by a reduction of oxygen in the blood.

Diaphragm
The dome-shaped sheet of muscle that separates the abdomen from the chest cavity. It is the major muscle of inhalation.

Dyspnea
Breathing that has become difficult or labored.

Emphysema
A disease characterized by the rupture of *alveoli*, caused by cigarette smoking. Symptoms include progressive *dyspnea*, cough, and impaired airflow when the person exhales.

Empyema
An accumulation of pus in a body cavity or in certain organs. Empyema in the *pleura* is a rare complication of lung infection.

Farmers' lung
An occupational lung disease affecting farm workers. *Hypersensitivity* develops upon exposure to certain molds or fungi that grow on hay or straw.

H-I

Hemoptysis
Coughing up of blood from the respiratory tract.

Histamine
A chemical released by certain cells in the body during an allergic reaction or inflammation that produces such symptoms as watery eyes, wheezing, and a runny nose.

Hypersensitivity
A reaction of the immune system to an *antigen*.

Hypersensitivity pneumonitis
Inflammation of the lungs caused by an allergic reaction to inhalation of dust containing certain animal or plant materials.

Hyperventilation
Abnormally deep or rapid breathing that occurs in heart diseases, central nervous system disorders, metabolic diseases, and anxiety.

Hypoventilation
A reduced breathing rate.

Hypoxia
A reduction in the oxygen supply to the body.

Influenza
A sometimes severe viral infection that causes cough, fever, headache, muscle aches, and weakness.

Intercostal muscles
Thin sheets of muscle between each rib that help to expand and contract the chest during breathing.

L-N

Laryngitis
Inflammation of the *larynx* that results in hoarseness.

Laryngoscopy
Examination of the *larynx* with a mirror or with a viewing tube called a laryngoscope.

Larynx
The organ in the throat that contains the vocal cords and produces voice sounds.

Lobar pneumonia
Lung infection confined to one lobe of a lung.

Mast cell
A cell that plays a role in the immune response.

Mediastinoscopy
Investigation of the *mediastinum* with a flexible endoscope inserted through an incision in the neck.

Mediastinum
The central part of the chest between the lungs containing the heart, *trachea*, esophagus, thymus gland, major blood vessels, lymphatic vessels, and nerves.

Mesothelioma
A tumor of the *pleura*. There is an increased incidence of mesothelioma in people exposed to asbestos fibers.

Newborn respiratory distress syndrome
Any condition in a newborn that interferes with the passage of oxygen from the air sacs in the lungs to the blood. It is usually caused by a deficiency in *surfactant*.

P

Pancoast's tumor
A rare form of lung cancer.

Percussion
A part of the doctor's examination in which he or she taps the chest and listens to the resonance of the sound produced.

Pharyngitis
Inflammation of the *pharynx*. The main symptom is a sore throat.

Pharynx
The passage that connects the back of the mouth and the nose to the esophagus and *trachea*; the throat.

Phrenic nerves
The principal nerves supplying the *diaphragm*.

Pickwickian syndrome
A disorder characterized by obesity, shallow breathing, excessive daytime sleepiness, *sleep apnea*, and heart failure. Most symptoms disappear with weight loss.

Pleura
A two-layered membrane. One layer lines the inside of the chest cavity and the other covers the outside of the lungs.

Pleural effusion
An accumulation of fluid between the two layers of the *pleura*.

Pleurisy
Inflammation of the *pleura*, usually caused by an infection in the lungs.

Pneumoconiosis
A group of lung diseases caused by inhalation of mineral dusts.

Pneumonectomy
A surgical procedure to remove an entire lung.

Pneumonia
Inflammation of the lungs that causes coughing and fever. It is usually caused by an infection.

Pneumothorax
A collection of air in the space between the two layers of *pleura*.

Pulmonary edema
A buildup of fluid in the lung tissue, usually caused by heart failure.

Pulmonary embolism
Obstruction of a pulmonary artery or one of its main branches by a blood clot.

Pulmonary fibrosis
Scarring and thickening of lung tissue. It may result from previous lung infection, as part of a *pneumoconiosis*, or for no known reason.

Pulmonary hypertension
Elevated blood pressure in the arteries supplying a person's lungs.

R

Respiratory arrest
Sudden cessation of a person's breathing.

Respiratory failure
A condition characterized by a buildup of carbon dioxide and a decrease in the level of oxygen in the blood. It is caused by such conditions as *pneumonia*, heart failure, or *emphysema*.

S

Silicosis
An occupational lung disease caused by inhaling dusts containing silica.

Sleep apnea
Periods of cessation of breathing, of 10 seconds or longer, during sleep.

Status asthmaticus
A life-threatening *asthma* attack.

Sternum
The breastbone.

Stridor
Noisy, high-pitched breathing caused by abnormal narrowing of the *larynx*.

Surfactant
A substance produced by certain lung cells that prevents the *alveoli* from collapsing during exhalation.

T-V

Thoracotomy
An operation in which the chest is opened.

Trachea
The windpipe.

Tracheotomy
Non-emergency surgery in which an opening is created in the *trachea*. A tube is usually inserted to keep the airway open.

Vagus nerve
A nerve with branches to the *larynx* and *trachea* along which messages travel from the brain to control swallowing, coughing, speech quality, and, in part, breathing.

W

Walking pneumonia
A mild case of *pneumonia* that does not require complete bedrest.

Wheeze
A whistling sound produced by breathing, caused by airway narrowing.

INDEX

Page numbers in *italics* refer to illustrations and captions.

Photograph sources:
Heather Angel/Biofotos Ltd 37; 43 (center left)
Ardea London Ltd 15; 114 (bottom left)
Art Directors Photo Library 83
Bart's Medical Picture Library 31 (bottom left); 131 (center)
Biophoto Associates 43 (top left); 79; 102
Collections 29
Colorific Picture Library 91
The Environmental Picture Library 50
Dr. S. Gwyther 74 (right); 134
Robert Harding Picture Library 110 (bottom left); 114 (top right)
The Image Bank 7; 34/35; 45 (bottom right); 49; 59; 86 (left); 94 (top left); 112 (bottom left); 113 (bottom left); 137 (right)
National Medical Slide Bank, UK 53; 88 (bottom left); 112 (bottom right); 129
The Photographers' Library 90

Pictor International Ltd 9; 41; 87
Science Photo Library 2 (top left); 21; 26; 31 (bottom right); 70 (center left); 72 (bottom left); 75; 76 (top right); 77 (top center); 77 (bottom); 80; 86 (bottom); 86 (top right); 113 (top left); 126; 137 (top left)
Shell UK 45 (top left)
Tony Stone Worldwide 2 (bottom left); 36; 110 (bottom right); 111 (bottom right)
John Watney Photo Library 138
Dr. J. Young 117; 125
Zefa 38; 78

Front cover photograph:
Dan Bosler, Tony Stone Worldwide

Commissioned photography:
Susannah Price   Amanda Carroll

Illustrators:
Tony Bellue
Karen Cochrane
David Fathers
Tony Graham
Andrew Green

Peter Massey
Coral Mula
Guy Smith
Lydia Umney
Philip Wilson
John Woodcock

Airbrushing: Janos Marffy

Index: Sue Bosanko

Reader's Digest Fund for the Blind is publisher of the Large-Type Edition of *Reader's Digest*. For subscription information about this magazine, please contact Reader's Digest Fund for the Blind, Inc., Dept. 250, Pleasantville, N.Y. 10570.